The Diabetic Foot

The Diabetic Foot

An illustrated guide to management

William Jeffcoate FRCP
Consultant Physician and Endocrinologist,
City Hospital, Nottingham, UK

and

Rosamund Macfarlane MA
Medical Research Assistant, City Hospital, Nottingham

with the assistance of
Susan Hirst AIMI
Senior Medical Photographer

CHAPMAN & HALL MEDICAL
London · Glasgow · Weinheim · New York · Tokyo · Melbourne · Madras

Published by Chapman & Hall, 2–6 Boundary Row, London SE1 8HN, UK

Chapman & Hall, 2–6 Boundary Row, London SE1 8HN, UK

Blackie Academic & Professional, Wester Cleddens Road, Bishopbriggs, Glasgow G64 2NZ, UK

Chapman & Hall GmbH, Pappelallee 3, 69469 Weinheim, Germany

Chapman & Hall USA, One Penn Plaza, 41st Floor, New York NY 10119, USA

Chapman & Hall, Japan, ITP-Japan, Kyowa Building, 3F, 2-2-1 Hirakawacho, Chiyoda-ku, Tokyo 102, Japan

Chapman & Hall Australia, Thomas Nelson Australia, 102 Dodds Street, South Melbourne, Victoria 3205, Australia

Chapman & Hall India, R Seshadri, 32 Second Main Road, CIT East, Madras 600 035, India

First edition 1995

© 1995 William Jeffcoate and Rosamund Macfarlane

Designed by Geoffrey Wadsley
Typeset in 10/12pt Palatino
Printed and bound in Hong Kong

ISBN 0 412 54410 5

A catalogue record for this book is available from the British Library

Contents

Preface   ix

Acknowledgements   x

1   Introduction   1

2   The normal foot   11
    Appearance and surface anatomy   13
    Bones and joints   13
        X-rays   13
    Blood supply   13
    Innervation   13

3   Pathogenesis of foot lesions   19
    Introduction   20
    Predisposition   20
        Factors which reduce resistance to trauma   21
        Factors which increase the likelihood of damage   24
        Factors which precipitate a foot lesion   26
        A break in the skin   26
        Factors which delay healing   27
        Impaired wound healing in diabetes   27
        Barriers to early referral and early assessment   29
        The place of education in foot care   30

4   Classification and description of foot ulcers   31
    Classifications of foot ulcers   32
        Meggitt/Wagner classification   32
        Nottingham classification   32
    Descriptions of foot ulcers   33
        Describing an ulcer in a referral letter   33
        Describing an ulcer in medical and nursing records   34

5   Infection in the diabetic foot   35
    Soft tissue infection — cellulitis   37
        Identification   37
    Bone infection — osteomyelitis   39
        Identification   39
        Charcot deformity and osteomyelitis   43
        Management of osteomyelitis   43
    Microbiology   43
        Identification   46
        Management of infection   48

6 Vasculopathy — **51**

Introduction — 52
Normal inflammatory process — 52
    Thrombosis — 53
    Mobilization of neutrophils and monocytes — 53
    Vasodilatation and new vessel formation — 53
    Epithelialization and organization — 53
Macrovascular disease — 53
    Atherosclerosis — 53
    Hypertension and hyperlipidaemia — 54
    Smoking — 54
    Oral contraceptives and hormone replacement therapy — 55
Microvascular disease — 55
Identification of ischaemia in the diabetic foot — 56
    Signs of chronic ischaemia — 57
    Typical lesions of the ischaemic foot — 57
Investigation of ischaemia — 59
    Examination of peripheral pulses by Doppler — 59
    Toe plethysmography — 60
    Transcutaneous oxygen tension — 60
    Duplex ultrasonography — 60
    Angiography — 60
Treatment of macrovascular disease — 63
    Angioplasty — 63
    Thrombolysis — 66
    Arterial surgery — 66
Skin grafting — 67
Other measures — 67

7 Neuropathy — **69**

Pathogenesis — 70
Types of peripheral neuropathy — 70
    Sensory neuropathy — 70
    Motor neuropathy — 71
    Proprioceptive loss — 73
    Autonomic neuropathy — 73
Recognition of neuropathy — 75
    Inspection — 75
    Examination — 76
Management of the neuropathic foot at risk of ulceration — 77
    Definition of the 'at risk' foot — 77
    Reducing abnormal pressure — 78
Management of neuropathic ulceration — 81
    Alleviation of pressure — 81
Neuropathic osteoarthropathy — Charcot joint — 82
    Pathogenesis — 83
    The process of diabetic neuropathic osteoarthropathy — 85
    Recognition — 85
    Investigations — 86
    Management of acute neuropathic osteoarthropathy — 87
    Management of chronic deformity — 87
    Prevention — 88

8	**Skin and nail conditions**	**89**
	Skin conditions associated with diabetes	90
	Dry skin	90
	Necrobiosis lipoidica diabeticorum	90
	Eruptive xanthomata	91
	Diabetic dermopathy	91
	Granuloma annulare	91
	Lichen planus	92
	Bullosis diabeticorum	93
	Hyperkeratosis from psoriasis	93
	Trauma	93
	Dermatitis artefacta	94
	Vasculitic and purpuric rashes	94
	Other skin conditions	94
	Mycological infections of the feet and toenails	95
	Tinea pedis	95
	Tinea unguium	97
9	**Chiropody**	**99**
	Skin care	100
	Nail care	100
	Callosities	102
	Corns	102
	Ulcers	102
	Neuropathic ulcers	102
	Neuroischaemic ulcers	103
	Amputation sites	103
	The place of chiropody in ulcer management	103
10	**Applications and dressings**	**105**
	The healing process	106
	Healing of ulcers in diabetes	107
	Principles of wound management	109
	Debridement of slough and eschar	109
	Cleaning	113
	Applications	113
	Dressings	114
	Compression bandaging	116
	Alleviation of pressure	116
	Psychological and social aspects of wound management	116
	Potentially adverse effects of dressings	117
	Summary	117
11	**Amputation and rehabilitation**	**119**
	Introduction	120
	When should amputation be considered?	120
	Localized surgery	121
	Major surgery	123
	The process of rehabilitation	126
	The perioperative phase	127
	Later rehabilitation	127
	Problems in the rehabilitation phase	129
	Outcome after amputation	130

12 Prevention of foot ulcers   **131**
  Education of people with diabetes   132
    The young and fit   132
    The older, fit person   132
    The patient whose feet are 'at risk'   133
    What to teach   135
    Adverse effects of patient education   136
  Education of the professional   136
    The general practitioner   136
    Nurses working in primary care   136
    Receptionists   137
    Chiropodists   137
    Doctors in hospitals   137
    Nurses in hospitals   137
  Assessment for the provision of fitted footwear   138
    Selection of patients for orthoses   138

13 Foot ulcers in perspective   **141**
  Prevalence of foot problems   142
    Ulcers   142
    Amputation   142
  Costs   142
    Costs of health and community services   142
    Costs to the patient   143
    Costs to the family and carers   143
  Inefficiencies in the management of foot lesions   143
  The role of the multidisciplinary clinic   143
    Coordination of care   143
    Education   144
    Research   144
    Failings of the multidisciplinary service   144
  The future   144
    Prevention of foot ulcers   144
    Coordination of care   144
    The St Vincent Declaration   144

**14 Practical guide to the management of lesions of the diabetic
    foot**   **145**
  General principles   146
  Suggested approaches to management of individual lesions   146
    Cases 1—16   147

Index   **163**

Preface

Lesions of the foot affect an estimated 7% of people with diabetes at some stage, and are one of the most feared complications of the disease. They can cause weeks and months of immobility and discomfort, and many never heal. Each year one diabetic in 250 will lose a leg by amputation. The cost of foot ulceration to both the individual and the Health Service is considerable. One reason why foot ulcers pose such an enormous problem is the large number of different factors that may contribute to their development and their perpetuation, but another concerns their management. Proper care requires the skills of a specialist multidisciplinary team and yet such a team is available in only a minority of towns. The majority of ulcers are treated by doctors and nurses who have had neither specific training nor experience — whether they work in primary care or as general physicians, geriatricians and surgeons in hospitals. It is for these professionals that this book is intended.

It is designed as a practical guide to the assessment and management of all types of lesion, and emphasis is placed also on the importance of prevention. To that end we have tended to offer simple, sometimes dogmatic, advice. In doing so, we accept that others may hold contrary views; this is a field in which there is much uncertainty — largely because it is one in which treatments have only rarely been evaluated by scientific study. Controlled trials are still needed in many areas to define optimal strategies for management.

This book is based on the experience we have gained in our own multidisciplinary clinic over the last 12 years. The clinic was established with the help of Emyr Wyn Jones and Ian Peacock, and has since been continued by many other medical and non-medical staff. To each and all we offer our thanks.

William Jeffcoate
Rosamund Macfarlane
Nottingham

Acknowledgements

This book could not have been produced without the help and inspiration of our colleagues and the cooperation of our patients, and we express our deep gratitude to them. We offer particular thanks to the following.

Susan Hirst, Senior Medical Photographer, City Hospital, Nottingham
Elisabeth Fletcher, Diabetes Specialist Nurse, City Hospital, Nottingham

Geoffrey Gilbert and staff, Audiovisual and Educational Services, University Hospital, Nottingham
Christopher Elston, Consultant Histopathologist, City Hospital, Nottingham (Figures 3.1, 3.7, 6.2, 6.3, 6.5, 6.7)
Alan English, Consultant in Rehabilitation, City Hospital, Nottingham and his staff (Figures 11.13, 11.14, 11.15, 11.16)
Roger Finch, Professor of Infectious Disease, University of Nottingham, Consultant Physician, CHN (Figures 5.27, 5.28, 5.29, 5.31, 8.16)
Mark Goodfield, Consultant Dermatologist, General Infirmary, Leeds (Figures 8.7, 8.19)
Stephen Haworth, Consultant Ophthalmologist, University Hospital, Nottingham (Figure 6.10)
Adrian Manhire, Consultant Radiologist, City Hospital, Nottingham (Figures 6.32, 6.33, 6.36(a), 6.42(a))
Donald Rose, Consultant Radiologist, City Hospital, Nottingham
John Tooke, Professor of Vascular Medicine, University of Exeter, Consultant Physician, Royal Devon and Exeter Hospital, Exeter (Figure 6.6)
Stephen Vernon, Senior Lecturer in Ophthalmology, University Hospital, Nottingham (Figures 3.6, 6.8)
John Ward, Professor of Diabetic Medicine, University of Sheffield, Consultant Physician, Royal Hallamshire Hospital, Sheffield (Figure 7.2)
Peter Wenham, Consultant Vascular Surgeon, City Hospital, Nottingham (Figures 6.16, 6.27, 6.28, 6.42(b), 11.1, 11.4, 11.8, 11.11)

and other non-medical members of our multidisciplinary team:
Nurses: Jean Moult and staff, Helen Sowter and staff
Plaster theatre: Ruth Hartley and Eileen Redgate
Chiropodists: Julia Williams, Alison Knowles, Jane Clarke, Alison Shone
Orthotist: Brian Biddulph
Occupational Therapist: Anne Rowe
Research Occupational Therapist: Marion Walker
Clerical and Secretarial: Sue Clark, Tracey Dickens, Sue Williams
Information and Computing: Neil Pound
Pharmacist: Catherine Truman

The extensive quotations in Chapter 1 are excerpted from information appearing in New England Journal of Medicine, 1934, 211, 16–20, 'The menace of diabetic gangrene', by Elliott P. Joslin.

We also thank John Macfarlane for the original idea.

1 Introduction

The management of ulcers on the feet of people with diabetes is one of the most neglected areas in clinical medicine. These lesions are common and their ultimate cost to the individual and the State is enormous, and yet few doctors and nurses receive specific training in their management. It is true that the options for management are limited, but in many cases the outcome can be improved by appropriate coordinated care and limbs can be saved. Although the issues of pathogenesis, treatment and prevention are discussed in detail in later chapters, it is pertinent to raise some of them in this introduction. We have chosen to do this by highlighting extracts from a review article published in 1934 in the *New England Journal of Medicine* by Elliott P. Joslin. This article was written before antibiotics were available and little more than a decade after insulin was discovered. It was a time when professional perceptions of diabetes and its long-term complications were very different from those of today. The style of scientific writing was also rather different.

The menace of diabetic gangrene
by Elliott P. Joslin, MD

...You may recollect that in the period investigated by Dr Hyman Morrison, 1895 to 1913, the deaths from gangrene amounted to 23 per cent and in a recent year I found that one-half of all the diabetic deaths in Boston Hospitals were due to gangrene. Boston makes a much better showing in 1933. Thus, there have been 261 deaths and of these, 37 or 14.1 per cent have resulted from gangrene and incidentally 34 or 13 per cent from diabetic coma.

> Note that this high incidence of death from ketoacidosis reflects the relatively recent introduction of insulin. Even though it was high by today's standards it should be remembered that ketoacidosis was almost invariably fatal 10 years earlier.

As a matter of fact, these percentages will be somewhat reduced because I find lacking in the death certificates furnished me, certificates for diabetic patients who died from cancer, tuberculosis and perhaps other diseases.

> To this day it remains difficult to define the contribution of diabetes to overall morbidity and mortality outcome, because mention of the disease is often omitted from official statistics. Previous studies of hospital activity analysis in UK have demonstrated a consistent 30–40% under-recording of diabetes, but our own recent data suggest that as many as 67% of events may be missed.

Lemann years ago pointed out that the mortality from gangrene among his private cases was eight times less than among the cases treated in the Charity Hospital in New Orleans.

> Joslin makes repeated reference to gangrene being an affliction of the poor and disadvantaged – something which is not true today, at least not in a country which provides comprehensive health care that is free at the point of delivery. It could be that this reflects the fact that those who do not have immediate access to a competent primary care physician will present later, and with more advanced disease.

Diabetic gangrene increases with the age of the patient and with the lengthening duration of the diabetes. The age at death of gangrene in the City of Boston group this year was above 60 years and the records of my own 81 deaths from gangrene since 1926 showed the average age to have been 67.5 years, the median age being practically the same, 67.7 years.

> These ages are remarkably similar to those of today. We have found that the mean age of amputation (almost universally for gangrene) is 66.7 years (men 63.6; women 72.3). This suggests that those who developed gangrene 60 years ago were very similar to those who develop it today. It also suggests that little has been achieved this century to affect the natural history of the prime cause of gangrene, which is arteriosclerosis.

Sex. The predominance of diabetes in females in middle life and onwards is well known but it is not so well known that this also holds for gangrene. Thus, of Boston's 37 gangrene deaths 24 were females and 13 males. Similarly in Dr Bolduan's recent compilation of the gangrene series in New York City there were 106 females and 53 males thus furnishing confirmation of the predominance of female diabetic deaths and indicating where our efforts should be focused.

> The predominance of females must have reflected the greater number of women with diabetes who reached this age. Presumably the men who would have been at risk died earlier from heart disease or lung cancer; cigarette smoking was far less common in women before the Second World War. In our experience over the last 10 years the number of men who undergo amputation is double that of women.

Season. Gangrene is less frequent in summer than in winter although in August, 1926 we had 12 cases of gangrene or infections of the feet at one time and the Boston statistics show that although we have had 37 fatal cases of gangrene in the city this year there were but a total of seven fatalities in the five months, July, August, September, October, and November. It is easy to understand why gangrene is more common in the winter because the circulation is less good and with cold feet sensation decreases and patients are more liable to burns and frost bites.

> There is no evidence of seasonal variation in the incidence of gangrene in UK today, although it is possible that the greater seasonal variation in climate in Boston contributed to these findings. It is worth noting, however, that Joslin refers here to **deaths** from gangrene and these deaths would have been largely the result of myocardial infarction or stroke – both of which **are** more common in winter months.

Furthermore, the feet are much less frequently bathed in the winter in the class of patients from which gangrene is largely recruited.

> Cleanliness and general foot care remain extremely important but would have been of even greater importance in the pre-antibiotic era. An injury would have been much more likely to become infected in a neglected foot, and infection is the main precipitant of gangrene in the ischaemic limb.

Onset of Gangrene Versus Onset of Diabetes Mellitus. Patients with onset of diabetes 30–39 years of age seldom develop gangrene and if they do it is postponed for 20.8 years as can be seen by the following table. When diabetes begins in the eighth decade, gangrene is apt to appear within 3.8 years on the average.

Table 1.1 Onset of gangrene versus onset of diabetes

Decade of onset	Number of cases	Duration of DM to beginning of gangrene
30-39	5	20.8
40-49	19	13.2
50-59	26	9.9
60-69	23	8.7
70-79	8	3.8

The younger the diabetic the longer the gangrene is postponed, but the diabetic had better remember this paraphrase of a Negro song, 'Gangrene will get you if you don't look out!'.

The Prevention of Gangrene. Diabetic gangrene is preventable in the over-whelming majority of cases, just as Priscilla White has demonstrated this to be true for diabetic children with cataracts and arteriosclerosis. (1.) Gangrene is overwhelmingly more common in the uncontrolled diabetic. I doubt if we see one patient in a hundred at the George F. Baker Clinic in which gangrene results from an embolus. Consequently, it has been forced upon me that gangrene is not Heaven-sent but is earth-born. The comparison between the incidence of gangrene in private and public patients as cited by Lemann shows the possibility of prevention. Fifty per cent of Eliason's cases of gangrene at the Philadelphia General Hospital did not even know they had diabetes. It certainly does pay to treat diabetes.

> Although the results of the Diabetes Control and Complications Trial (DCCT) trial published in 1993 did not include cardiovascular end-points, few physicians doubt that its conclusions can be extrapolated both to macrovascular disease and to non-insulin-dependent diabetes. Close control from the point of onset of diabetes is likely to reduce the incidence of all its complications.

The methods the average doctor is using today are far superior to older methods. We should be encouraged rather than discouraged and press our modern type of treatment upon the patient more and more. We are not aggressive enough in our treatment of diabetes. Dr. F.M. Allen has rightly said that the surest way to produce gangrene is to keep patients alive but only half treat them.

> Dr F. M. Allen may have been unfair. It is possible that it was not the poor control that facilitated the onset of gangrene, but the greater longevity.

Anything which will improve our treatment of the diabetics will tend to postpone the premature aging of the patients; in other words it will defer arteriosclerosis and thus avoid the great cause of gangrene.

(2.) Cleanliness is the second weapon we have to prevent gangrene. Unless there is trauma the clean patient almost invariably avoids gangrene. I cannot speak enthusiastically enough of the cleanliness which many patients show, but with poor people the opportunities for keeping clean are not favorable and they simply don't realize the necessity of doing so. Thus, at the hospital we always talk cleanliness and emphasize the importance of each patient being treated in the Beauty Parlor for Diabetic Feet even though he does not need to do so.

(3.) A history of trauma can nearly always be elicited from the patient. Burning the feet with a hot water bag, electric pad or chemical heater is about the most common injury, but a close second are injuries which come from new shoes, or their imperfect linings and ill-fitting old shoes.

> The first sentence of this paragraph would appear to contradict the points emphasized in the one which preceded it.

> Nothing has changed. Injuries from hot-water bottles, fires and shoes remain among the commonest precipitants.

In our directions for patients we emphasize all these points.

Epidermophytosis furnishes an easy mode of entrance for organisms, because of the frequent fissures which accompany that quite universal infection of the feet.

> Tinea pedis is not 'universal' but remains a very important cause of skin ulceration, and hence acts as a precursor to secondary bacterial infection.

(4.) Perhaps the best preventive measure of all which we have at the hospital is the exhibition to new-comers of a few patients who have had gangrene and amputations of a leg or a toe. These gangrene patients are a cheerful and courageous group. Visiting diabetics cannot help drawing useful lessons from the causes of their gangrene but also from the good spirits which they show.

> The question of educational methods is discussed in Chapter 12. We do not usually involve those who have suffered some of the ravages of diabetes to bring home the message, but perhaps we should.

Medical Treatment. The medical treatment of the diabetic patient with gangrene is simple, because the patient is under absolute control and is willing to do anything to save his extremity. Furthermore, the diabetes is usually mild in character, as was recognized by Naunyn.

> The whole question of close glycaemic control during the management of established foot ulceration remains unstudied. Since the process of healing is critically dependent on microvascular function and on resistance to infection, both of which are compromised by hyperglycaemia, it seems reasonable to conclude that we should all make greater efforts to achieve normoglycaemia in those with ulcers than we do at present. Maybe this should receive as much emphasis as it does, for example, in the management of diabetes through pregnancy.

Exercise is the mainstay of any diabetic and as soon as active infection subsides we promote this through help of a physiotherapist and with dumb-bells, pully weights and various measures. The pre-gangrene cases often use a Buerger board and that for an hour three times a day gives ample exercise for many of the older people.

Insulin is used freely, remembering that it is safer to give small doses often than large doses once a day to elderly people whose hearts are vulnerable; and practically all patients with diabetic gangrene have sclerosis of the coronary arteries.

> The only preparation available at that time was neutral (or soluble, short-acting) insulin. There were no orally active agents.

Soon the insulin can be decreased from three to two times a day, often to once a day and quite often omitted, but I think our custom now is to give insulin a little more freely than formerly, even if the urine is sugar-free, provided the blood sugar reaches 0.20 (200 milligrams) per cent.

> 200 mg/100 ml is equivalent to about 11 mmol/l. In other words, they were achieving far closer control than many of us do with our affected non-insulin-dependent patients today.

We use insulin decidedly more rather than less with our gangrene patients. However, we are very cautious about overdosage with insulin with elderly people and particularly so at the time of operation....

Indications for Operation. By operation it is understood that usually amputation of an extremity is meant. These indications are as follows:

1. Gangrene in a painful, pulseless foot.
2. Pain in a pulseless foot which is not relieved within two weeks by rest in bed, Buerger's exercises and other medical measures.
3. Osteomyelitis. Here a toe alone may be amputated. Indeed an additional toe may be sacrificed merely to secure adequate drainage.
4. Recurrent ulcers in a callus.
5. Extensive infections which necessitate a guillotine operation.

> The indications remain much the same, although amputation should be rarely undertaken nowadays for neuropathic ulceration.

The surgeon occasionally can break the rule and amputate a toe in the absence of a pulsating dorsalis pedis artery and secure a good result. In such instances the collateral circulation is particularly abundant and the foot warm. No instrumental methods for the determination of the circulation are equal to palpation of the blood vessels, the observation of the ischaemic or cadaveric color of the foot on the bed, and of rubor when the feet are hung down out of bed for three minutes, and the persistence of pain following two weeks in a horizontal position.

> These remain the cardinal clinical signs of critical ischaemia, although the place of 'instrumental methods' is far more important today because of the options available for vascular reconstruction.

Dead bone can be detected by a probe, before it is visualized by X-ray.

> This remains true. Osteomyelitis may be apparent clinically several weeks before it is obvious on X-ray.

Hospital stay has been gradually shortened. In a recent summary it was 47 days for minor infections and 52 days for minor lesions due to defective circulation, in contrast to 41 days for major operations due to infections and 38 days for major operations due to impaired circulation. Even the non-operative cases remained in hospital for an average of 19 days. Surgical treatment is time-consuming and expensive. It costs far more to save a toe than a leg.

> Data from Switzerland in the early 1980s provide an interesting contrast to these figures. In Geneva the mean duration of in-patient stay was reported as 26 days for a distal amputation, but 111 days for a below-knee amputation.

Sad to relate it is the exception for the diabetic who has gangrene or an infection of a leg which demands amputation to survive more than three years after discharge from the hospital.

> Overall survival following amputation remains poor. The details are given in Chapter 11, but in our experience less than 50% survive 3 years after amputation of a leg. Women do worse than men, but the average age of women at amputation is greater (72 versus 64 years).

Prior to operation no insulin is given as a routine unless obviously indicated by the individual case. Our object in curtailing insulin is to avoid the possibility of hypoglycaemia during the operation. No preoperative medication is given for the amputation cases and this applies to morphine, atropin and tetanus antitoxin. Wounds are sewn up tight and not drained. The preliminary use of perfringins antitoxin has not been found to be necessary. There have been but two cases of gas bacillus infection in our diabetics at the Deaconess in six years. Ointments and moist dressings are avoided in gangrene cases. Following operation the patient is placed in bed with a Balkan frame with handles from the upper bars so as to facilitate moving about in bed and thus obtaining exercise. It also facilitates nursing care. A heavy woolen sock is placed on the remaining foot so that it will be protected from cold, heat, and pressure on the bed. Similarly pillows rather than rings are used to keep the remaining heel off the bed.

> This essential piece of secondary prevention is frequently forgotten in hospitals today. Heavy woollen socks, or some other form of protection for the other heel, should be invariably used.

During convalescence every inducement is made to teach the patient to walk with a peg leg before he leaves the hospital. We are far more interested in the patient having a peg leg than an artificial leg. At home he may not make an effort to walk or the cost of an artificial leg may delay his attempt.

The financial aspect of gangrene is serious. The medical treatment of gangrene during weeks or months in home or hospital is far more expensive than early surgery. It is likewise more wearing on the patient's nerves. Subsequently patients regret the postponement of their operation and returning to hospital advise other patients to be operated on earlier. So many of these late cases come to me in financial straits and so few pay my surgical colleagues anything, that I am almost ashamed to look the latter in the face. An infected or gangrenous foot before it is healed costs, in my opinion, at least $300, quite apart from medical, surgical or special nursing fees or loss of wages.

Delay in the recognition of the seriousness of an infection of the foot and delay in reporting to a physician are analogous to the delay in detection of early tuberculosis.

> This last section mainly refers to two different themes: procrastination which merely delays an inevitable amputation, and procrastination which leads to deterioration of the lesion. While the first of these is debatable, and a case must be considered for early surgery in everyone, it is the latter which causes greater concern today. Delayed referral for expert assessment may lead to unnecessary deterioration of some ulcers.

Even when the doctor is consulted early, it is easy to temporize not only for those medical men unaccustomed to cases of gangrene, but for those of us who see a great many cases. I have the greatest sympathy with practitioners who are called upon to care for these patients, because over and over again we ourselves, who see so many in the hospital, delay too long in advising operation.

Death from gangrene to-day is usually the result of procrastination on the part of the physician.

> Avoidable death is now uncommon, but avoidable gangrene is not as uncommon as it should be.

2 The normal foot

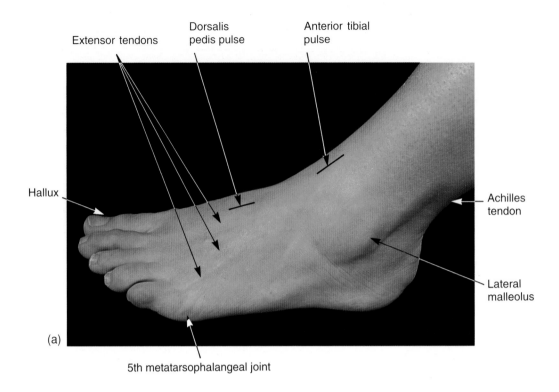

(a)

Extensor tendons

Dorsalis pedis pulse

Anterior tibial pulse

Hallux

Achilles tendon

Lateral malleolus

5th metatarsophalangeal joint

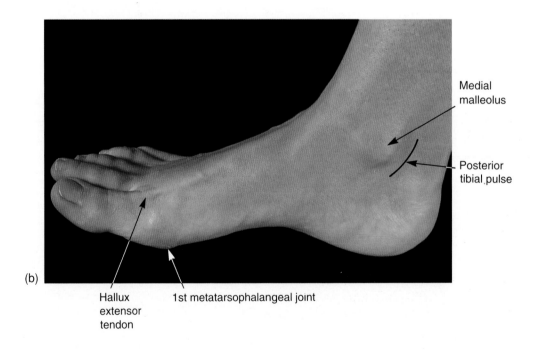

(b)

Medial malleolus

Posterior tibial pulse

Hallux extensor tendon

1st metatarsophalangeal joint

Figure 2.1 Some of the main landmarks on **(a)** the dorsal surface and **(b)** the medial aspect of the foot.

APPEARANCE AND SURFACE ANATOMY

The skin of the healthy foot is elastic but resilient. It should not show signs of scaliness, dryness or brittleness, nor should it be thin and shiny. Plantar skin is about twice as thick as that on the dorsum, is tougher and moves less readily over deep structures. The points which take the greatest pressure – the heel and the metatarsal heads – are protected by fatty pads beneath the skin. The heel is further protected by the specialized honeycomb structure of the deep tissues.

The arch of the foot is maintained by the plantar fascia and by the action of the muscles of the foot. When the normal balance between these muscles is affected by peripheral neuropathy, the arch of the foot is either lost (flat foot), or it becomes exaggerated (pes cavus). In either case this leads to the exertion of abnormal pressure loading – particularly under the metatarsal heads and under the tips of the toes. The skin responds to this increased pressure by forming callus.

The main surface markings of the foot are illustrated in Figure 2.1.

BONES AND JOINTS

The foot is made up of 27 bones, 19 muscles and 32 joints, which are arranged to form the longitudinal and transverse arches and provide a base which is strong enough, and resilient enough, to take the whole weight of the body. The bones are divided into three basic groups: the tarsals, the metatarsals and the phalanges (Figure 2.2). In normal standing the weight is shared equally between the pads under the metatarsal heads and the heel. About a third of the weight is taken by the pad under the first metatarsal head.

During walking the weight is taken first on the point of the heel ('heel strike'). It is then transferred smoothly to the outer aspect of the sole and the metatarsal heads of the second to fifth toes. It then shifts medially to the ball of the foot (first metatarsal head) and the body is propelled forward by flexion of all the metatarsals, and of the big toe ('toe off'). This smooth transfer of forces is lost when the foot loses its normal plantar arch, or the ligaments and soft tissues become less elastic. The result is that some parts of the sole take increased pressure and therefore become liable to neuropathic ulceration. This is most likely to occur over the second and third metatarsal heads, and the big toe.

X-rays

Three views are used in routine clinical practice. The anteroposterior (AP) (Figure 2.3(a)) view shows details of the metatarsals and phalanges, but most of the tarsal bones are blurred. The oblique view (Figure 2.3(c)) shows further details of the metatarsals, as well as the navicular and cuneiforms. The calcaneum and talus are best seen on the lateral view (Figure 2.3(b)). Exaggeration of the plantar arch with pes cavus, and associated clawing of the toes, is also best seen on the lateral view.

BLOOD SUPPLY

The aorta divides at the level of the fourth lumbar vertebra to form the common iliac arteries on each side. The internal iliacs supply the pelvic tissues while the external iliac supplies the leg. At the level of the inguinal ring it is called the common femoral and this then divides to form the profunda femoris and the main artery to the lower leg, the superficial femoral artery (Figure 2.4(a)).

The superficial femoral becomes the popliteal at the level of the knee and this then divides to form three main branches in the calf: the anterior tibial, the posterior tibial and the peroneal (Figure 2.4(b)). The anterior tibial becomes the dorsalis pedis (Figure 2.5(a)) while the posterior tibial passes behind the medial malleolus to divide into the medial and lateral plantar arteries (Figure 2.5(b)).

The dorsalis pedis divides into the arcuate artery and the perforating branches – which pass between the metatarsal heads to anastomose with the deep plantar arch of the lateral plantar artery. Branches from all of these contribute to the paired digital arteries which supply each toe. Figure 2.6 demonstrates the effect of these details in clinical practice: thrombosis of both digital arteries causes gangrene of the whole toe, whereas thrombosis of only one leads to necrosis of only half the toe.

INNERVATION

Detailed knowledge of the distribution of the peripheral sensory nerves to the lower leg and foot is not of much value in clinical practice. Although neuropathy is a common complication of diabetes, it tends to be diffuse and to affect all distal nerves to a similar extent. Loss of sensation is found in a 'stocking' distribution and is not confined to the distribution of any one nerve. The territories of the major cutaneous nerves are shown in Figures 2.7 and 2.8.

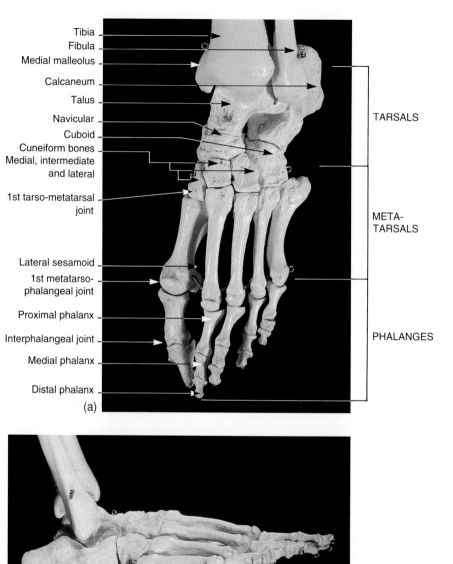

Tibia
Fibula
Medial malleolus
Calcaneum
Talus
Navicular
Cuboid
Cuneiform bones
Medial, intermediate
and lateral
1st tarso-metatarsal
joint

TARSALS

META-
TARSALS

Lateral sesamoid
1st metatarso-
phalangeal joint
Proximal phalanx
Interphalangeal joint
Medial phalanx
Distal phalanx

PHALANGES

(a)

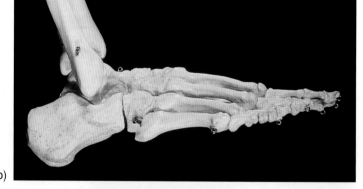

(b)

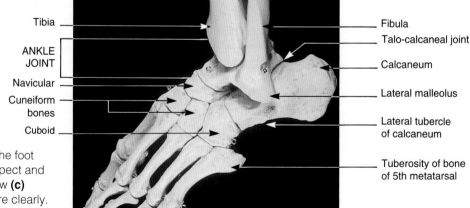

Tibia

ANKLE
JOINT

Navicular
Cuneiform
bones
Cuboid

Fibula
Talo-calcaneal joint
Calcaneum
Lateral malleolus
Lateral tubercle
of calcaneum
Tuberosity of bone
of 5th metatarsal

Figure 2.2 The bones of the foot seen from **(a)** the dorsal aspect and **(b)** the side. An oblique view **(c)** shows the tarsal bones more clearly.

(c)

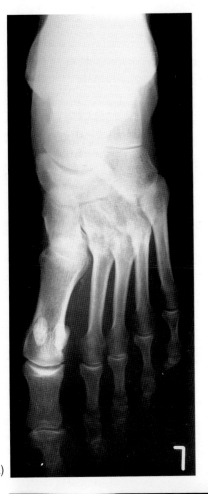

(a)

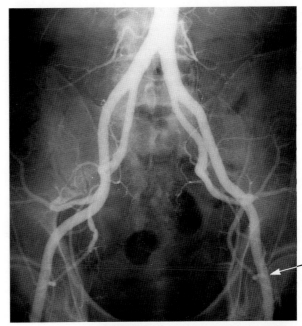

Common femoral artery

(a)

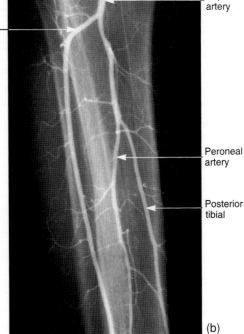

Popliteal artery

Anterior tibial artery

Peroneal artery

Posterior tibial

(b)

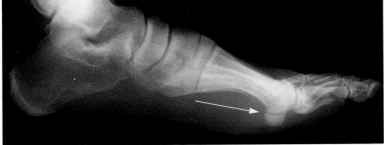

(b)

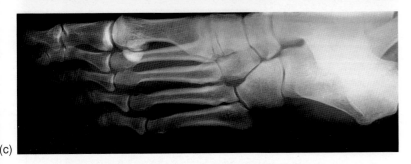

(c)

Figure 2.3(a) The AP view is best for the metatarsals and phalanges. **(b)** The lateral view shows the calcaneum and talus. One or two sesamoid bones (arrowed) may be seen; they are embedded within the flexor tendons of the hallux. **(c)** The oblique view shows the metatarsals, as well as the navicular and cuneiforms.

Figure 2.4(a) The main blood supply to the leg is derived from the superficial femoral artery, which is itself derived from the common femoral. **(b)** The popliteal divides into three branches – the anterior tibial, the posterior tibial and the peroneal – at a point below the knee called the trifurcation. The quality of flow in these vessels is commonly called the 'run-off'.

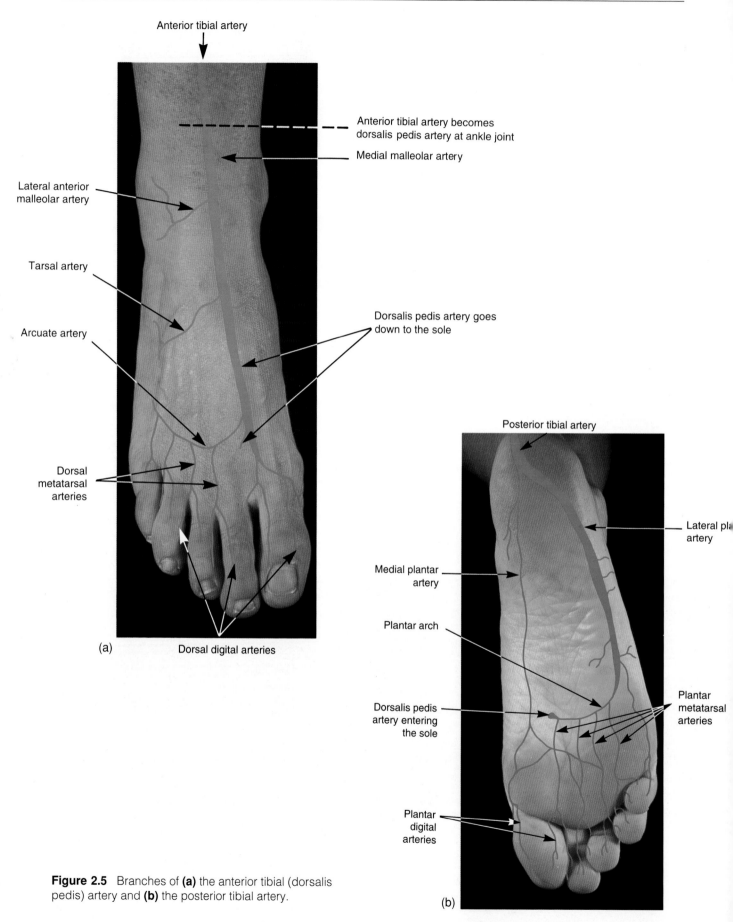

Anterior tibial artery

Anterior tibial artery becomes
dorsalis pedis artery at ankle joint

Medial malleolar artery

Lateral anterior
malleolar artery

Tarsal artery

Arcuate artery

Dorsalis pedis artery goes
down to the sole

Dorsal
metatarsal
arteries

Dorsal digital arteries

(a)

Posterior tibial artery

Lateral pl
artery

Medial plantar
artery

Plantar arch

Dorsalis pedis
artery entering
the sole

Plantar
metatarsal
arteries

Plantar
digital
arteries

(b)

Figure 2.5 Branches of **(a)** the anterior tibial (dorsalis pedis) artery and **(b)** the posterior tibial artery.

Figure 2.6 Thrombosis of the digital arteries leads to gangrene of the toe. When both the medial and lateral digital arteries are occluded, the whole toe becomes black, but it is possible for the blood supply on one side to be preserved while the other is occluded, as seen here.

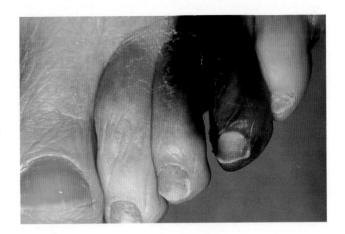

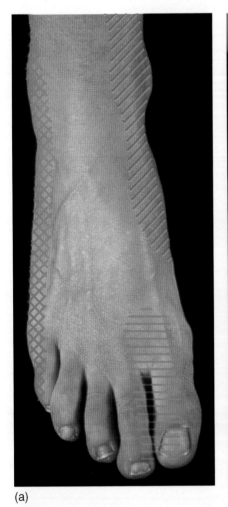

(a)   (b)

Figure 2.7 Cutaneous nerves on **(a)** the dorsum of the foot and **(b)** the sole.

Saphenous nerve		Medial calcaneal nerve
Sural nerve		Medial plantar nerve
Deep peroneal nerve		Lateral plantar nerve
Superficial peroneal nerve		

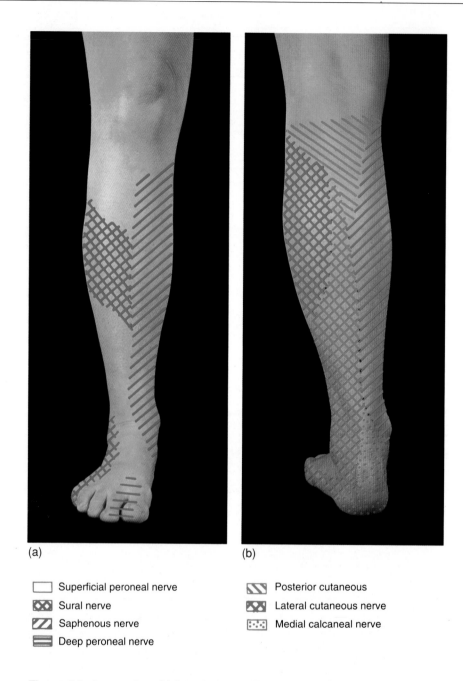

(a)   (b)

Superficial peroneal nerve		Posterior cutaneous	
Sural nerve		Lateral cutaneous nerve	
Saphenous nerve		Medial calcaneal nerve	
Deep peroneal nerve			

Figure 2.8 Innervation of **(a)** the front and **(b)** the back of the shin.

3 Pathogenesis of foot lesions

INTRODUCTION

Foot ulcers are common in the older diabetic and community surveys have shown that some 7% of them will have one at some stage. They occur because of diabetes itself, the complications of diabetes and the complications of advancing age. However, these various factors not only predispose a person to the development of an ulcer but also contribute to its perpetuation. In other words, an ulcer on the foot of a person with diabetes is less likely to heal quickly, more likely to become infected and to spread, and therefore more likely to result in amputation. Thus the pathogenesis of these lesions needs to be considered under three headings:

1. **predisposition** – the factors which put a certain individual 'at risk';
2. **precipitation** – the event which leads to an actual break in the skin, i.e. to ulceration;
3. **perpetuation** – the factors which delay healing and lead to complications.

PREDISPOSITION

Certain factors predispose an individual because they lead to changes in the tissues of the foot which make them less resistant to trauma and infection. Others actually make trauma and infection more likely. These are listed in Table 3.1.

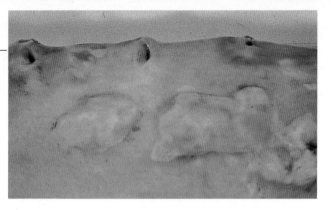

Figure 3.1 The aorta opened at post-mortem to demonstrate a large atherosclerotic plaque partly occluding the lumen.

Table 3.1 Factors which predispose the foot to ulceration in diabetes mellitus

Factors which reduce the resistance of the tissues to trauma

- Macrovascular disease: atherosclerosis, male gender, smoking
- Microvascular disease
- Autonomic neuropathy

Factors which increase the likelihood of trauma

- Motor neuropathy
- Sensory neuropathy
- Limited joint mobility
- Other complications of diabetes: visual impairment
- Other complications of growing old: unsteadiness, immobility, fires, hot water bottles

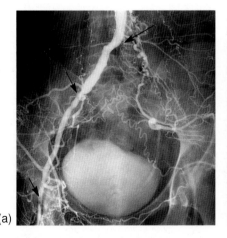

(a)

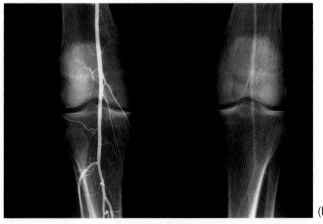

(b)

Figure 3.2(a) The aortogram of a woman with diabetes who had smoked all her adult life. She had gangrenous changes in both feet. The X-ray shows complete occlusion of the common iliac on the left (large arrow), as well as stenoses at the origin of the right external iliac and within the right superficial femoral (small arrows). There are numerous collateral vessels indicating that some of the obstructions have been present for a long time. She died of a myocardial infarction. **(b)** Angiogram in the same patient, showing reduced flow of contrast down the left leg as a result of the obstruction of the common iliac artery.

Factors which reduce resistance to trauma

MACROVASCULAR DISEASE

This refers to atherosclerosis, which narrows the large and medium-sized arteries to the leg and foot (Figures 3.1 and 3.2(a)). The reduction in delivery of oxygen and nutrients renders the whole foot relatively ischaemic and hence less able to maintain the normal integrity of the tissues (Figure 3.2(b)). Since the forces exerted on the joints, ligaments and skin during walking are enormous, there is a constant need for tissues to regenerate and this is limited by the presence of ischaemia.

There are obviously a number of factors which increase the likelihood of macrovascular disease, including those listed below.

Male gender (Figure 3.3):

Macrovascular disease is more common in men and men develop foot ulcers at an earlier age. The mean age of amputation in men is almost 10 years less than in women.

Cigarette smoking (Figure 3.4):

All forms of smoking increase the risk of macrovascular disease. It is very unusual for young insulin-dependent diabetics to develop problems with their feet unless they smoke.

MICROVASCULAR DISEASE

Diabetes is also associated with abnormalities of the smaller vessels – the arterioles, capillaries and venules. They are affected in three ways.

1. Thickening of the basement membrane which encircles the endothelium (Figure 3.5) leads to reduced transfer of nutrients across the cell wall

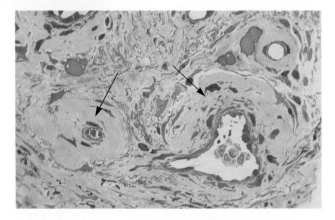

Figure 3.4 Cigarette smoking constitutes the greatest avoidable risk of atherosclerosis.

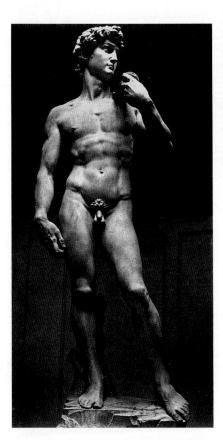

Figure 3.3 Men are more likely to develop macrovascular disease than women (reproduced by kind permission of Phaidon Press from *Michelangelo: Paintings, Sculptures, Architecture* by L. Goldscheider).

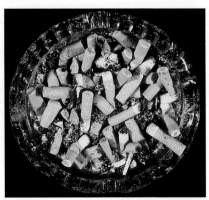

Figure 3.5 The basement membrane which surrounds the endothelial cells of capillaries is thickened in diabetes (arrowed). The cause of the thickening is not known but it results in defective transfer of nutrients from the capillary to the tissues.

and also reduced ability of the vessel to dilate as part of the normal protective process of inflammation.

2. Thrombosis of capillaries occurs because the thickened basement membrane causes them to be rigid and the red blood cells are less able to squeeze through. Other factors may contribute to hypercoagulability in diabetes, but the net effect is capillary closure, and this further exacerbates the ischaemia of the tissues (Figure 3.6).

3. Abnormal shunting of blood occurs as a result of loss of innervation of arterioles and venules. The integrity of tissues is normally maintained by diverting blood to areas where it is most needed, and this is achieved by appropriate dilatation and constriction of small blood vessels (Figure 3.7). Diabetics with peripheral neuropathy may lose the innervation of these vessels and hence they are unable to shunt blood where it is needed.

The subject of macrovascular and microvascular disease is covered in more detail in Chapter 6.

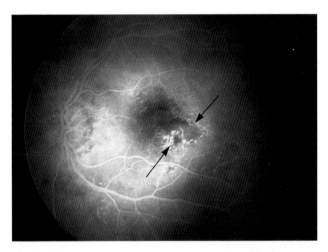

Figure 3.6 This fluorescein angiogram of the retina demonstrates areas (arrowed) in which the capillaries have shut down as a result of thrombosis. Equivalent changes take place in the small blood vessels of the foot.

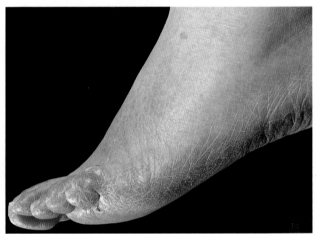

Figure 3.8 The relative ischaemia caused by autonomic neuropathy may leave the skin dry and flaking, and this is made worse by the associated loss of sweating, which reduces the resistance to infection.

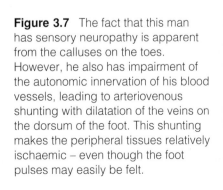

Figure 3.7 The fact that this man has sensory neuropathy is apparent from the calluses on the toes. However, he also has impairment of the autonomic innervation of his blood vessels, leading to arteriovenous shunting with dilatation of the veins on the dorsum of the foot. This shunting makes the peripheral tissues relatively ischaemic – even though the foot pulses may easily be felt.

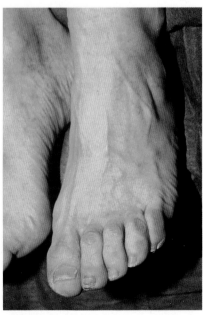

AUTONOMIC NEUROPATHY

Diabetes affects all the nerve fibres to the foot (motor, sensory and autonomic) but it is the loss of the autonomic innervation that renders the foot more susceptible to any trauma to which it is exposed. Loss of the motor and sensory supply simply makes the foot more likely to be exposed to trauma (see below). The autonomic supply is essential for shunting the blood to areas of need (see Microvascular disease, above) and is also important for the maintenance of normal skin structure. The details of this nutritive effect are not known beyond the fact that sweat glands are innervated by autonomic fibres and loss of normal sweating leaves the skin of the foot dry, liable to

crack and less resistant to trauma. The protective antimicrobial effect of sweat is also lost (Figure 3.8).

CHARCOT NEUROPATHIC OSTEOARTHROPATHY

This subject is dealt with in detail in Chapter 7, but it is relevant to mention it here because the process results in abnormal thinning of bones, which makes them liable to fracture in response to forces that would not break normal bones (Figure 3.9). Once the bones become disorganized, the joints are destabilized and the process of destruction becomes progressive.

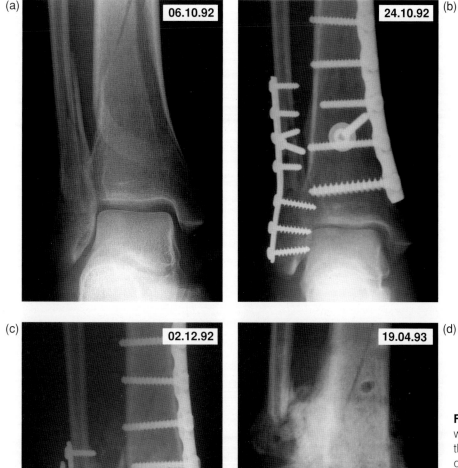

(a) 06.10.92 (b) 24.10.92 (c) 02.12.92 (d) 19.04.93

Figure 3.9 This man was in his 30s when he developed spiral fractures of the tibia and fibula while he was dancing. The fracture may have resulted from abnormal thinnning of the bones because of unrecognized Charcot neuropathic osteoarthropathy. The progressive destruction of the bones and joint which followed may have been caused by infection introduced at surgery, but it is equally likely that it simply represents progression of the osteoarthropathy. He lost his leg.

Factors which increase the likelihood of damage

MOTOR NEUROPATHY

When motor nerves are affected, there is weakness and wasting of the muscles in the foot. The muscle wasting is not obvious in the foot, but it can be assumed that any person who has motor neuropathy affecting the hands will have it in the feet as well (Figure 3.10).

This leads to imbalance between the flexors and extensors of the toes, leading to loss of the normal plantar arch, which may become either flattened or, more commonly, exaggerated. The resultant 'clawing' (Figure 3.11(a)) results in abnormal pressure being exerted on the metatarsal heads, the tips of the toes and the knuckles, and these then become sites at which pressure necrosis and ulceration may

occur (Figure 3.11(b)). This process is described in more detail in Chapter 7.

SENSORY NEUROPATHY

If patients are unaware of discomfort, they will not realize when the foot is threatened. Thus, they might have a small stone, or even a thumb tack (Figure 3.12) in their shoe and not feel it, or might burn the tips of their toes as they snooze in front of the fire (Figure 3.13). Choosing new shoes is especially difficult because they cannot tell if the shoes are pinching or not: all shoes feel comfortable to someone with anaesthetic feet.

Painful peripheral neuropathy

Other people have a peripheral sensory neuropathy which results in pain, rather than numbness. Painful peripheral neuropathy causes a persistent burning, aching, tingling feeling which is often worse in bed at night and relieved by both putting the leg out of the bed and by letting it hang down. Painful peripheral neuropathy is associated with a reduced risk of ulceration – presumably because it makes people more aware of their feet.

LIMITED JOINT MOBILITY

Diabetes causes abnormalities of connective tissue: the incorporation of carbohydrate into protein by a non-enzymatic process (glycosylation) renders collagen stiff and less flexible. In addition, there are complex changes in the structure and function of extracellular matrix proteins which are only dimly understood. These changes restrict joint mobility leading, for example, to the increased incidence of frozen shoulder in diabetes. In the foot, their main

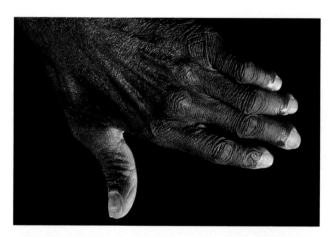

Figure 3.10 Wasting of the small muscles of the hand indicates motor neuropathy. The wasting is not so obvious in the foot.

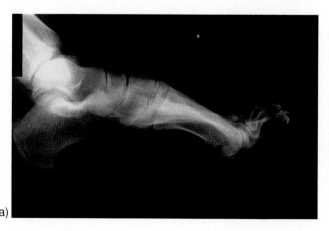

(a)

Figure 3.11(a) Clawing of the toes as a result of motor neuropathy. **(b)** Exaggeration of the plantar arch with clawing of the toes leads to excessive pressure being

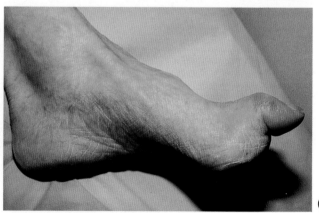

(b)

exerted at certain points: under the metatarsal heads, on the knuckles and tips of the toes. These are the areas most likely to ulcerate.

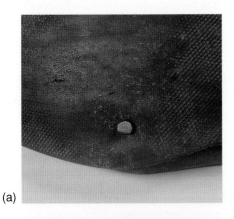

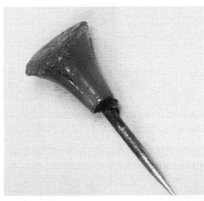

(a)

(b)

Figure 3.12 Thumbtack unnoticed in the sole of a shoe worn by a diabetic to the foot clinic. The wear on the top of the thumbtack suggests that it had been present for some time. It was unnoticed because of sensory neuropathy and caused a penetrating ulcer under the fifth metatarsal head which took 3 months to heal.

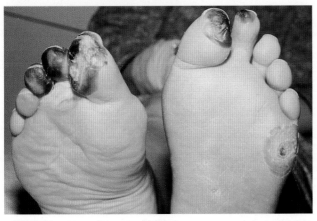

Figure 3.13 Burns on the tips of the toes caused by dozing in front of the fire.

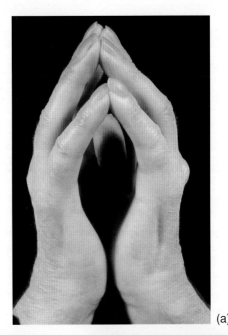

(a)

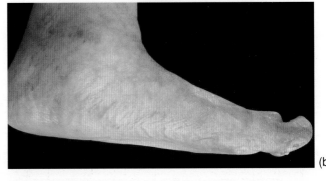

(b)

effect is to limit flexibility of the toes. As normal walking is dependent largely on the extension and then flexion of the big toe, limited movement of the metatarsophalangeal and interphalangeal joints critically alters the distribution of forces – leading to ulceration, usually of the hallux (Figure 3.14).

OTHER COMPLICATIONS OF DIABETES

Immobilization from stroke, heart attack or other illness will put the person at risk of ulceration of the heel (Figure 3.15). A hypoglycaemic attack may mean that a person is unconscious on the ground for a period of time, and hence also liable to pressure ulceration.

COMPLICATIONS OF GROWING OLD

Foot ulcers occur most frequently in the elderly; ulcers which do badly are most likely in those with peripheral vascular disease and significant vascular

Figure 3.14(a) Limited joint mobility is caused by glycosylation of collagen and other connective tissue. The joint capsules are rendered less flexible, as demonstrated in this illustration of the 'prayer sign': a person who has severe limited joint mobility is unable to press the hands flat together. This man suffered a bilateral amputation for associated peripheral vascular disease. **(b)** Limited joint mobility in the foot makes the hallux more rigid and less able to dorsiflex to absorb the forces exerted during walking. It is commonly associated with ulceration of the hallux, as illustrated here.

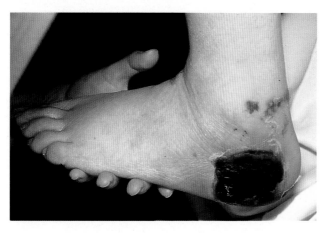

Figure 3.15 Immobilization from any illness puts the ischaemic foot at very great risk. Although it is sometimes said that 'heel ulcers never heal', this is not strictly accurate; about half of them do. This illustration is of an ulcer on the heel of the man whose hands are shown in Figure 3.14(a). He had been immobilized following amputation of his other leg.

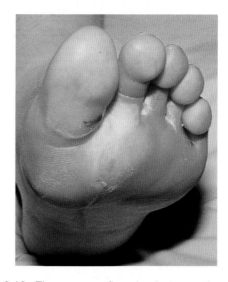

Figure 3.16 Tinea causes fissuring between the toes and this acts as a portal for pathogenic bacteria. In this case the infection is contained, but the effects can be catastrophic if the foot is ischaemic.

disease is more prevalent with advancing age. Old people are also less well able to care for the feet and are increasingly dependent on others to do it for them. Their feet may therefore be neglected or subjected to more clumsy care. They are more liable to stumbles and accidents, more likely to use hot water bottles (which may damage the skin) and more likely to sit in front of the fire. They are more likely to be immobilized through ill-health and hence predispose to pressure sores.

FACTORS WHICH PRECIPITATE A FOOT LESION

Sometimes a problem (e.g. arterial embolus, Charcot neuropathic arthropathy) arises in the diabetic foot without there being any actual ulcer, but in the vast majority of cases it is a break in the skin which is the precipitating factor.

A break in the skin

TINEA

Tinea causes flaking and fissuring of the skin between the toes. It occurs in people of any age. It causes little problem in the young, but in the older person with ischaemic feet the break in the skin can be the portal of entry for pathogenic bacteria. It may lead to loss of the leg (Figure 3.16).

TRAUMA

Most traumatic injury to the foot is accidental, and thus largely unavoidable. This includes blisters, burns and scalds (Figure 3.17), abrasions, perforating injuries and clumsy nail clipping. All too often the trauma concerned is the pressure exerted on the heel during a period of immobilization in hospital.

Trauma to the neuroischaemic foot

Accidental trauma is the result of abnormal forces acting on the foot, but ulceration can also result from the normal forces exerted during everyday standing and walking. This occurs if the foot is both ischaemic and anaesthetic (the so-called 'neuroischaemic' foot) and pressure sores are then liable to occur at sites of normal lateral and vertical pressure, usually from shoes. This is the cause of the multiple small scabs which may be seen on the knuckles of the toes (Figure 3.18). Ischaemic toes are also less resistant to vertical shearing forces exerted on the skin on the sides of the toes, and this results in 'kissing ulcers' (Figure 3.19).

Trauma to the neuropathic foot

Trauma is also responsible for the development of the classical, plantar neuropathic ulcer (Figure 3.20): the increased force exerted under the head of the metatarsals leads to pressure necrosis of the skin and underlying tissues. This subject is discussed in greater detail in Chapter 7.

FACTORS WHICH DELAY HEALING

Impaired wound healing in diabetes

Ulcers on the foot of a diabetic are worrying because they are slow to heal and quick to become complicated. The reasons why they are slow to heal are discussed in Chapters 6 and 10, and the complication concerned is nearly always infection (Chapter 5).

Once an ulcer is infected, healing is delayed still further and underlying ischaemia is worsened: arteries narrowed by atherosclerosis will become occluded by thrombosis if surrounded by inflammation (Figure 3.21).

While these various pathological processes are discussed in detail elsewhere, it is relevant to highlight the fact that the deterioration is not always

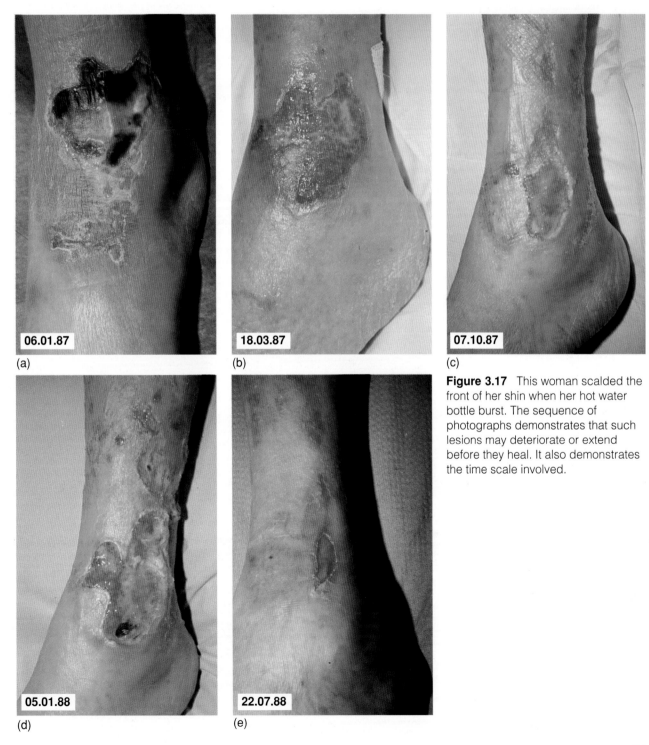

(a) 06.01.87   (b) 18.03.87   (c) 07.10.87

(d) 05.01.88   (e) 22.07.88

Figure 3.17 This woman scalded the front of her shin when her hot water bottle burst. The sequence of photographs demonstrates that such lesions may deteriorate or extend before they heal. It also demonstrates the time scale involved.

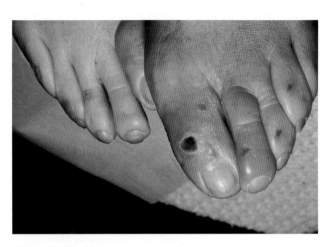

Figure 3.18 The occurrence of multiple, scabbed, superficial ulcers is a sign of ischaemia. The integrity of the skin is so far reduced that it breaks down in response to the normal pressures exerted by footwear, or even by bedclothes.

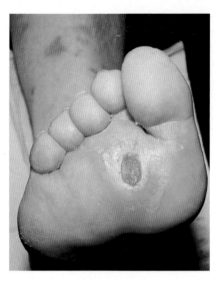

Figure 3.20 Excessive pressure under the metatarsal heads results in the build-up of callus, which is unnoticed because of associated sensory neuropathy. The effect of the callus is to increase the forces on the deeper tissues; pressure necrosis results in the development of the classical 'neuropathic' plantar ulcer shown here.

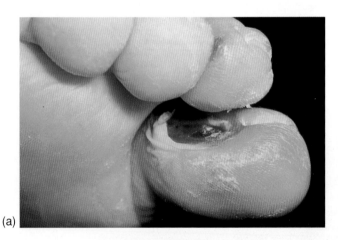

(a)

Figure 3.19 Vertical shearing forces may ulcerate the skin between the toes. These 'kissing' ulcers may persist for months. The drawing in **(b)** shows that 'kissing' or 'neuroischaemic' ulcers between the toes may result from either lateral pressure (left) or from vertical shearing forces (right).

(b)

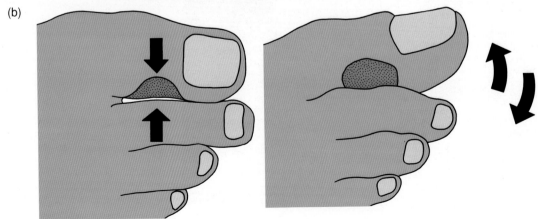

inevitable and it may be preventable by early referral and early expert assessment. The problem is that the structure of health care services is such that it is commonplace for delays to occur and these delays may sometimes result in the loss of a limb.

Barriers to early referral and early assessment

PATIENT FACTORS

The patient may be unaware of an ulcer and/or may be unaware of its significance. Patients may be unaware of its existence because of reduced visual acuity from cataract, retinopathy or glaucoma, or because they cannot bend down to inspect their feet. It is possible that people who clean their feet less often will also be slow to recognize an ulcer, but Joslin's belief that gangrene occurred largely in the poor and dirty seems out of proportion today: 'the clean person almost invariably avoids gangrene (and)

with poor people the opportunities for keeping clean are not favorable'.

However, patients may also be unaware of the significance of a sore that they have and may simply hope that it will 'go away'. Such blind optimism is part of human nature. Patients may also delay seeking help because they are embarrassed or ashamed that they have a foot problem. Such guilt may sometimes be worsened by an educational process which overemphasizes that it is the patient's own responsibility to prevent ulcers (Chapter 12).

Social deprivation

If poverty and social deprivation (Figure 3.22) are associated with the development of more severe foot ulceration, it would seem that this relates not so much to cleanliness as to other factors.

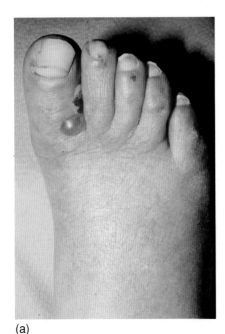
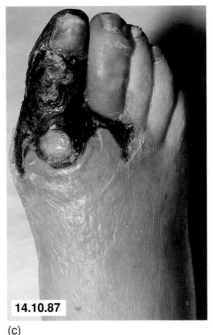
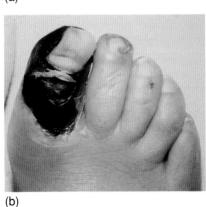
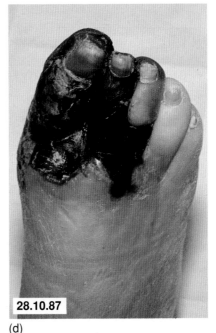

Figure 3.21(a) Tinea has been complicated by secondary infection but the cellulitis is not obvious because the foot is ischaemic. The threatening signs are the blackness between the toes and the blistering. Furthermore, the dusky blueness of the hallux suggests that it may become gangrenous. **(b)** Established gangrene of the hallux in the same foot 6 days later. **(c)** The paired digital arteries of the hallux have been occluded by cellulitis in the forefoot, and the second toe is also looking bluish. **(d)** Progression of the process in **(b)**, with the second and third toes both becoming necrotic.

(a)

(b)   (c)   14.10.87   (d)   28.10.87

Figure 3.22 If ulcers of the foot, and especially ulcers that are complicated, are associated with poverty and social deprivation, it is most likely to be because of lack of education and of lack of ready access to effective primary care (reproduced by kind permission of Nottingham County Council Leisure Services from the Local Studies Library).

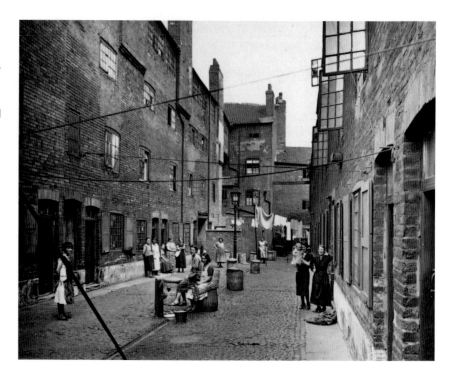

It may be partly the result of an increased prevalence of complications from, for example, smoking and partly the result of delay in seeking professional help. In other words the poor present late and with a greater likelihood of losing the leg because they are not aware of, or do not have easy access to, a good primary health care system.

DELAYS IN PRIMARY CARE

Doctors and nurses in primary care may also be unaware of the significance of a foot lesion and of how it should be best managed. They may be unaware of specialist services available in the town or may, like the patient, be reluctant to refer because of an ill-defined sense of guilt. Thus, they might feel that a foot ulcer is a 'simple' problem that they ought to be able to get better themselves. Paradoxically, such delays may be greater in better practices with more resources and a greater sense of independence. There is a fear that such delays will become more likely if the current changes in the NHS in the UK increase the effective barriers to specialist referral.

General practitioners will often delegate management to a nurse who then feels that it is her responsibility to induce healing and is naturally reluctant to admit defeat. Chiropodists also will sometimes feel reluctance to refer foot problems to specialists – referring, as they must, through a general practitioner who they might believe (and sometimes with justifi-

cation) knows less of the issues than they do, to a hospital doctor who they suspect (and often with equal justification) knows just as little. The problem for chiropodists is not made easier by the managerial isolation in which they seem to work in most towns.

DELAYS IN SECONDARY CARE

Delays are equally prevalent in hospitals, with patients often being managed primarily by junior staff or by teams whose main expertise is in another field. There may be a degree of unawareness of the multidisciplinary specialist skills available – even in the same hospital – and some degree of reluctance to use them. Just as in primary care, there are barriers to efficient cross-referral, with some physicians having difficulty in obtaining angiography and/or surgical advice as quickly as might be needed. In a town in the UK in which there are two multidisciplinary foot care services centred on the two specialist diabetes clinics, it has been calculated that three-quarters of amputations for diabetes are performed without their being consulted.

The place of education in foot care

The incidence of foot ulceration and of lower limb amputation will be reduced by continuing effort at education – education of the patient but, of even greater importance, of the professional too (Chapter 12).

4 Classification and description of foot ulcers

Descriptions are used to improve communication: to convey to someone else the exact nature of an ulcer. Classifications tend to be used more for scientific analysis of numbers seen, outcome, etc. While classifications are used only by those with a specialist interest in the field, descriptions are used by everybody.

CLASSIFICATIONS OF FOOT ULCERS

Meggitt/Wagner classification

The only classification which is used at all widely is that originally described by Meggitt and Wagner (Figure 4.1).

Lesions are coded 0–5 depending on their severity. It has the great advantage of simplicity, but the great disadvantage of being imprecise. Thus, a lesion classified Grade 0 (with no break in the skin) might represent accumulation of callus, a blister or critical ischaemia. On the other hand, one graded 3 might indicate either osteomyelitis in a well-perfused foot with little risk of amputation or extensive cellulitis in an ischaemic foot, for which major surgery is the only option.

Nottingham classification

We have evolved a more detailed classification, based on key aspects of pathogenesis and management (Table 4.1).

Thus, ulcers are divided into three broad groups: infection, ischaemia and neuropathy, and each of these groups is subdivided as shown. While it is

Table 4.1 Nottingham classification of foot ulcers

Infection

1. Cellulitis
2. Osteomyelitis

Ischaemia

1. Symptomatic ischaemia without an ulcer
2. Painless scabbed lesions of the skin
3. Gangrene
4. Persistent unhealing ischaemic lesions
5. Ischaemic heel ulcers
6. Blisters

Neuropathy

1. Ulcers with surrounding callus over an area of increased pressure
2. Neuropathic ulcers under the calcaneum
3. Ulcers caused by unnoticed trauma
4. Acutely evolving Charcot deformity

recognized that many lesions have mixed causes (involving, for example, both infection and ischaemia, or both ischaemia and neuropathy), they are allocated to the group which best reflects immediate management. In this way a foot affected by osteomyelitis would be classified under infection even though it may also be neuropathic (Figure 4.2); treatment with antibiotics is the first priority.

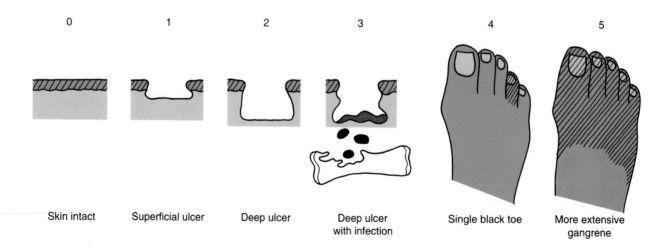

| 0 | 1 | 2 | 3 | 4 | 5 |

Skin intact   Superficial ulcer   Deep ulcer   Deep ulcer with infection   Single black toe   More extensive gangrene

Figure 4.1 The Meggitt/Wagner classification of foot lesions is the one which is most widely used. It is simple, and has the advantage of grading severity: a lesion may pass from one classification to another as it either heals or deteriorates. Its main disadvantage is that it is imprecise and non-specific.

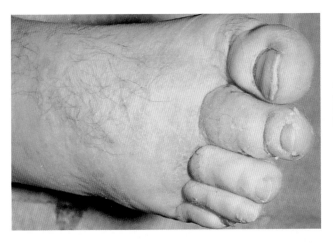

Figure 4.2 The second toe is swollen and distorted as a result of osteomyelitis, and treatment with antibiotics is therefore the most important aspect of immediate management. The infection gained access to the bone through a pre-existing neuropathic ulcer under the second metatarsal head (not shown).

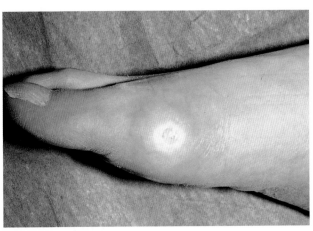

Figure 4.3 Although this man has clinical evidence of both vasculopathy and neuropathy (and there is a classical 'neuroischaemic' ulcer over the first metatarsophalangeal joint), it is the vasculopathy which poses the greatest risk. Angiography should be considered sooner rather than later.

On the other hand a non-infected superficial ulcer over the first metatarsophalangeal joint of someone with both peripheral vascular disease and neuropathy would be classified as ischaemic because prime consideration should be given to undertaking angiography (Figure 4.3).

Those which are predominantly neuropathic require neither antibiotics nor angiography, and the mainstay of management is the removal of inappropriate pressure from the sore.

The subdivision of these groups is based on the broad categories of ulcer that occur. Each subdivision can be further divided for research purposes, but this is of little value in clinical practice.

DESCRIPTIONS OF FOOT ULCERS

The problem is that foot ulcers come in so many different forms that there is no simple way of describing them in writing. People use vague terms such as 'diabetic foot' or 'ulcer' – terms which convey little of the severity of the lesion or the urgency needed in management. A picture gives the best impression because we rely largely on visual pattern recognition in clinical practice; the use of words can become quite long-winded. For this reason a verbal description has to be structured: it has to contain key elements in order to convey the maximum information in the minimum space. Ideally, it should include the following:

1. site;
2. side (left or right);
3. size (area or depth);
4. severity;
5. sepsis (i.e. clinically obvious infection);
6. source (some idea of the cause).

There are a number of other features which are also helpful, including the presence of pain, duration of the lesion and whether or not the foot is ischaemic. If these characteristics (the '6S' system) form the basis of a referral, the recipient will gain a good impression of the nature of the problem and of how s/he needs to respond.

Describing an ulcer in a referral letter

A doctor, nurse or chiropodist wishing to describe the ulcer in Figure 4.4 might therefore put the following in a referral to a specialist centre: 'The patient has a nasty looking infection on the right foot, which extends through the whole forefoot. The foot is ischaemic and is starting to go dusky-blue. I first saw it this morning but she thinks it started to become discoloured 3 days ago: it looks as though it may be caused by secondary infection of tinea between the toes.'

The expert reading this would be able to conjure a mental image of the problem immediately, and would realize that the foot was at risk, required urgent treatment with antibiotics and, possibly, angiography.

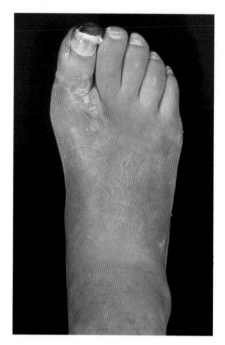

Figure 4.4

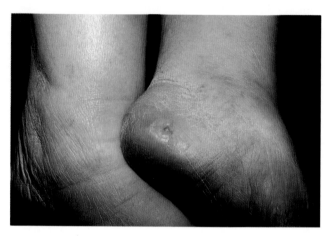

Figure 4.5

Alternatively, the lesion in Figure 4.5 might be described as follows: 'This man has a small, clean-looking ulcer on the inside of his left heel which is exquisitely painful. There doesn't seem to be any cellulitis and although I can't feel any foot pulses, the feet do not look particularly ischaemic. It all started when he was in bed following a stroke 6 months ago.'

Describing an ulcer in medical and nursing records

There is no substitute for a photograph or a drawing – no matter how crudely it is done. Thus, the lesions shown in Figures 4.4 and 4.5 might be recorded as in Figure 4.6.

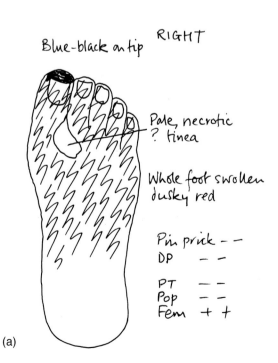

(a)

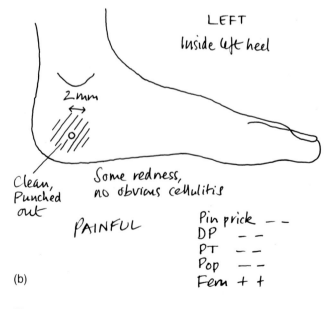

(b)

Figure 4.6 Drawings to document the features of the lesions shown in **(a)** Figure 4.4 and **(b)** Figure 4.5.

5 Infection in the diabetic foot

When infection occurs in the diabetic foot, it is nearly always secondary to a pre-existing break in the skin. Thus, infection is the consequence of ulceration and not the cause. The only exception to this rule is infection of either the skin or the nail with tinea pedis or with *Candida albicans*.

The break in the skin which predisposes the foot to infection may be caused by any of a number of processes including accidental trauma (Figure 5.1), ingrowing toenail (Figure 5.2) and ulceration from pressure necrosis (Figure 5.3). Indeed, the break caused by tinea pedis may itself act as a portal of entry for more pathogenic organisms (Figure 5.4).

The nature and severity of the infection depends partly on the nature of the infecting organism(s) and partly on the blood supply. In general, infection of the well perfused foot leads to either classical cellulitis or to osteomyelitis; infection in the ischaemic foot leads to gangrene.

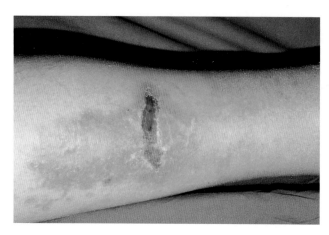

Figure 5.1 Rubbing by a work boot on the back of this man's shin caused an abrasion which became secondarily infected.

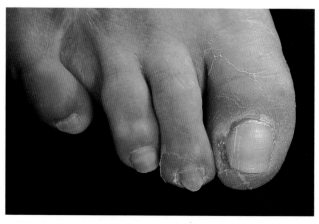

Figure 5.2 Ingrowing toenails, as here on the big toe, can create a break in the skin that acts as a portal for infection.

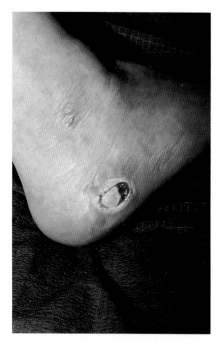

Figure 5.3 (left) This necrotic ulcer started on the outside of the heel when the patient was immobilized in bed following a stroke. When the foot is ischaemic, as in this case, pressure ulcers can arise even when every effort is made to reposition the patient frequently.

Figure 5.4 (right) Tinea pedis causes a break in the skin – leading to spreading cellulitis. When the blood supply to the foot is poor, cellulitis may be enough to precipitate gangrene. The purplish discoloration of the great toe in this case was a threatening sign: the patient went on to have a below-knee amputation.

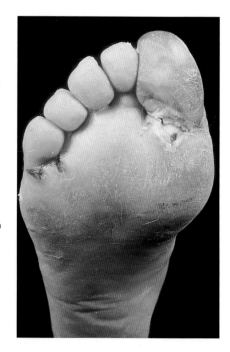

SOFT TISSUE INFECTION – CELLULITIS

Identification

Infection of soft tissues results in classical signs of inflammation: *rubor* (redness) (Figure 5.5), *calor* (warmth), *tumor* (swelling) (Figure 5.6) and *dolor* (pain). However, classical inflammation occurs only if there is a good blood supply and, since the blood supply is often poor in diabetes, it follows that the signs of infection are not always obvious.

Redness and swelling tend to be less obvious in ischaemic feet, although there may be other clinical signs. Thus, there might be an exudate – in which the infection is either obvious (Figure 5.7) or less so (Figure 5.8). Smell is typical of anaerobic organisms and these tend to thrive in more devitalized tissue (Figure 5.9). X-rays may show evidence of gas-forming organisms (Figure 5.10) which are usually either anaerobic bacteria or coliforms. Life-threatening gas gangrene from *Clostridium perfringens* is excessively rare.

Some people develop subacute or chronic infection of the soft tissues of the shin (Figure 5.11). Sometimes this infection seems to arise in an area affected by necrobiosis lipoidica (Figure 5.12), but it can be

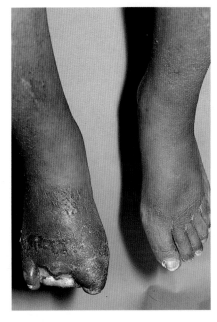

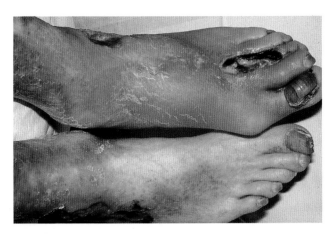

Figure 5.5 Redness (*rubor*) of the foot is a sign of infection.

Figure 5.6 Puffy swelling (*tumor*) following amputation of digits on the right foot is a sign that infection has been caused by bacteria entering through the unhealed wound.

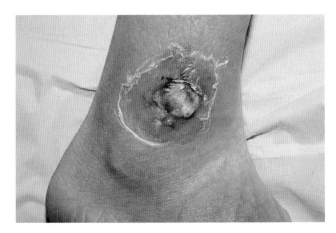

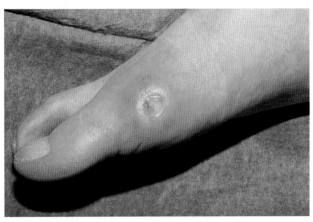

Figure 5.7 Exudate on a shin wound, which is obviously infected.

Figure 5.8 Sometimes the exudate over an infected ulcer is thin and almost clear.

impossible to tell without undertaking a skin biopsy. This is rarely done, however, because the result does not affect management. The organisms most often involved in such subacute infection are Gram-positive cocci, such as staphylococci and streptococci, and anaerobic bacteria.

Pain may be a symptom of active infection in a foot which is not otherwise obviously inflamed. A small clean ulcer may persist painlessly for many months over a bony prominence, but when it is painful it is usually infected (Figure 5.13).

The onset of pain may indicate that infection has penetrated to an interphalangeal or metatarsophalangeal joint beneath the superficial ulcer – without any evidence of surrounding bone infection. Having said that, great care must be taken to determine that the pain is actually localized to the ulcer and surrounding tissue and not caused by coincidental painful peripheral neuropathy. The fact that infection is associated with pain is surprising because such feet are nearly always affected by sensory neuropathy and are otherwise numb.

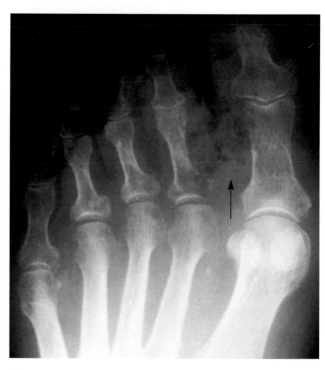

Figure 5.10 The presence of gas in the tissues may be apparent on plain X-rays (arrowed). It indicates the presence of gas-forming organisms such as anaerobes or coliforms.

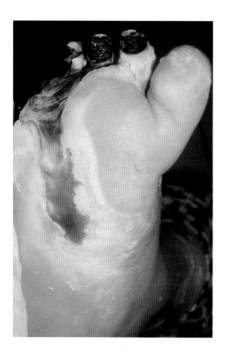

Figure 5.9 When there is extensive devitalized tissue, the lesion is likely to be infected by a number of different organisms, including anaerobic bacteria. The presence of anaerobes is likely if the infected foot smells, or if the patient has a fever.

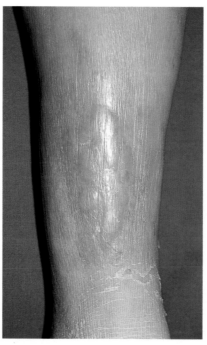

Figure 5.11 Subacute infection of the shin is usually caused by Gram-positive cocci and by anaerobes.

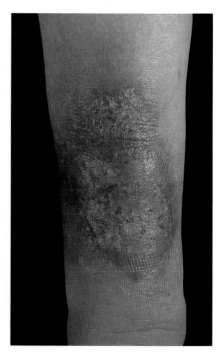

Figure 5.12 Subacute infection of the shin may be indistinguishable from necrobiosis lipoidica diabeticorum in its acute stages. Sometimes the infection occurs in an area of necrobiosis.

Another clinical sign of soft tissue infection is the occurrence of black digits – either single or multiple. When a patient develops gangrene of a toe in this way (Figure 5.14), it is usually possible to trace the following sequence of events.

There will have been a pre-existing break in the skin which has acted as the portal of entry for pathogenic bacteria. The inflammation caused by these organisms may not be clinically obvious, but it is this which leads to the thrombosis of the paired digital arteries of the toe. In other words, the gangrene – which looks like the primary event – is actually the result of infection.

BONE INFECTION – OSTEOMYELITIS

Osteomyelitis of the diabetic foot is a condition with relatively specific clinical signs, confirmed by the characteristic appearances on plain X-ray. However, the processes involved in the development of osteomyelitis in the diabetic foot are different from those involved in classical, haematogenous osteomyelitis: neither the clinical nor the radiological signs are the same. The bone infection which occurs in diabetes occurs, once again, as a secondary event: the organisms gain access to bone through a pre-existing ulcer in the skin, rather than via the blood stream.

The organisms most commonly involved in the development of osteomyelitis are Gram-positive cocci (notably streptococci and *Staphylococcus aureus*) and anaerobes. Presumably the requirement of aerobic cocci for a well oxygenated microenvironment is the reason why osteomyelitis usually occurs in well perfused feet, most typically as secondary infection of a neuropathic ulcer. Infection of less well perfused feet leads not to osteomyelitis but to gangrene.

Identification

When bone infection is obvious, the diagnosis is easy. It is primarily clinical, but confirmed radiologically.

CLINICAL SIGNS

The infection nearly always affects the toes, either the metatarsals or the phalanges. The affected toe is podgy and swollen like a sausage and typically has a thickened red, brawny skin (Figure 5.15(a)). There may or may not be pus. If it is present, it may be discharging from multiple sinuses (Figure 5.16). The lesion is painless, and the person has no signs of systemic infection.

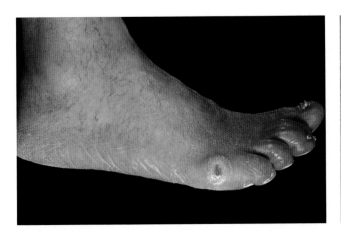

Figure 5.13 When chronic ulcers become painful, they are usually secondarily infected. If the blood supply to the foot is poor, there may be no sign of inflammation or other clue to the presence of infection. The pain may indicate involvement of the underlying joint. If so, movement of the toe will make the pain worse, and may make a bleb of exudate appear.

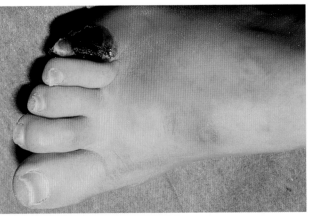

Figure 5.14 When a patient presents with a single black toe adjacent to an area of cellulitis, it is usually thought that it is the gangrene of the toe which is the primary lesion and that the cellulitis is secondary. More often, however, it is the infection which causes the gangrene.

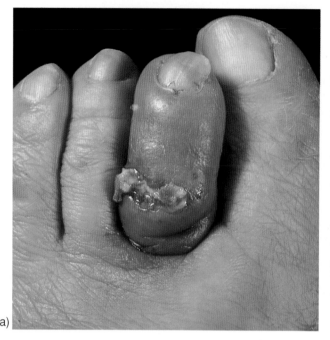

(a)

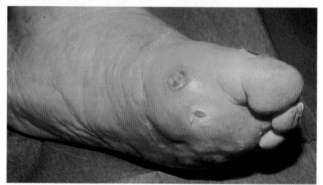

(b)

Figure 5.15 Osteomyelitis most commonly affects the toes, and when it does, the appearances are usually unmistakable. **(a)** The toe becomes brawny-red and sausage-shaped, with or without evidence of discharging pus. **(b)** The X-ray appearances of osteomyelitis in the same toe; the bone cortex is interrupted and the bone is fragmented.

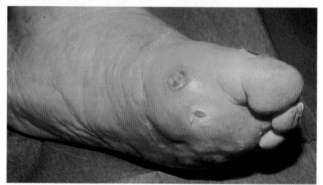

Figure 5.16 Pus discharging from multiple sinuses in a toe affected by osteomyelitis.

(b)

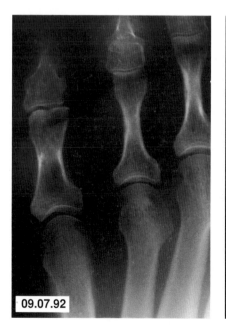

09.07.92

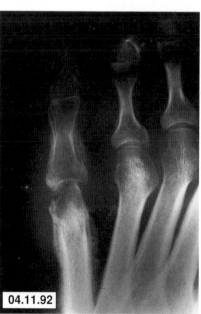

04.11.92

Figure 5.17(a) This man was treated for osteomyelitis of the fifth toe on the basis of the clinical appearance – even though there were no clear confirmatory signs on X-ray. The radiological signs were apparent 4 months later. **(b)** The typical X-ray appearances of osteomyelitis with loss of the metatarsal head and marked subperiosteal new bone formation in the same foot. By this time the lesion was clinically resolving.

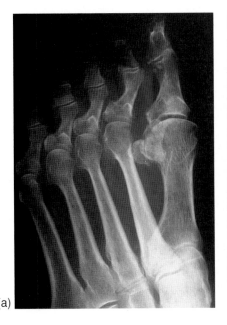

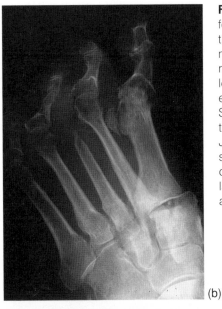

(a)

(b)

Figure 5.18(a) This lady was treated for clinically apparent osteomyelitis of the left hallux even though there was no radiological confirmation in this X-ray taken in July 1992. A labelled leucocyte scan might have helped to establish the diagnosis at this stage. She also had gangrene of the third toe. **(b)** The same foot X-rayed in June 1993, when there were clear signs of resolving bone infection, with destruction of the first metatarsophalangeal joint. The third toe has been amputated.

(a)

(b)

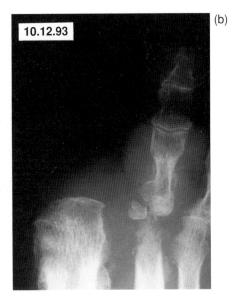

05.06.93

10.12.93

Figure 5.19(a) Both phalanges of the hallux are infected: the cortex is interrupted and the bone structure is destroyed. There is also gas in the soft tissues – suggesting involvement with anaerobic bacteria. The second toe seems normal. **(b)** An X-ray of the same foot. The hallux has been amputated but the second toe is now involved and the metatarsophalangeal joint has been destroyed.

RADIOLOGICAL SIGNS

The cardinal sign on plain X-ray is interruption of the bone cortex, with or without fragmentation of bone (Figure 5.15(b)). The X-ray changes often lag behind the clinical signs, sometimes by several months (Figures 5.17 and 5.18). Sequential X-rays may show the sequential involvement of different toes (Figure 5.19).

While clinical appearance and plain X-ray remain the main basis for diagnosis, the use of labelled leucocyte scanning is increasing; the labelled cells concentrate at sites of bone infection. It may be hard to distinguish osteomyelitis from uncomplicated infection of overlying soft tissue, but it may be of great value in differentiating it from Charcot osteoarthropathy (Figure 5.20).

In contrast, three-phase bone scanning with labelled diphosphonate – in which persistence of isotope at 2–3 hours indicates increased bone turnover – will usually differentiate osteomyelitis from cellulitis, but not from Charcot arthropathy.

OTHER INVESTIGATIONS FOR OSTEOMYELITIS

Measurement of either erythrocyte sedimentation rate (ESR) or C-reactive protein (CRP) is of no value. Indeed, it is worth noting that the ESR is nearly always extremely high (60–120 mm/h) in any foot ulcer which has been present for more than a week or

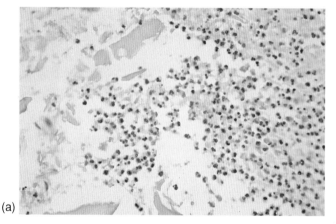

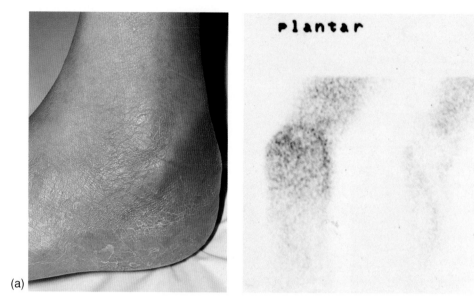

(a)

(b)

Figure 5.20(a) This man presented with progressive painful swelling of the heel after he tripped over a kerbstone. The skin had not been broken at any time. Although the appearances are typical of osteomyelitis, they are in fact the result of Charcot's neuropathic osteoarthropathy. The scan **(b)** shows some increased uptake of technetium-HMPOA-labelled leucocytes in the soft tissues – but none of the increased uptake in bone which would be expected in osteomyelitis.

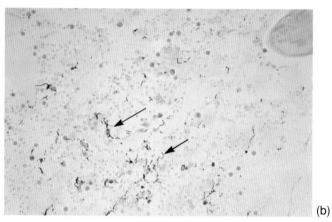

(a)

(b)

Figure 5.21(a) Histological specimen obtained from a foot amputated because of generalized gangrene and without clinical or radiological evidence of osteomyelitis. The appearances are typical of bone infection, with destruction and inflammatory cell infiltrate – emphasizing that bone biopsy alone is insufficient for the diagnosis of the syndrome which behaves clinically as osteomyelitis. **(b)** Higher-power view of the same specimen, showing abundant bacteria, including streptococci (arrowed).

two. Alkaline phosphatase will be high, reflecting increased activity of osteoblasts.

It is often said that bone biopsy is the gold standard for defining the presence of bone infection, but it is nearly always impractical. Many doctors are reluctant to undertake any unnecessary surgical procedure in the foot of a person with diabetes – in case there is delayed healing of the wound. Moreover, the findings on biopsy may not be as specific as is usually thought. Thus, the appearances in Figure 5.21 were obtained from the bones of a foot amputated for gangrene; they show classical features of osteomyelitis – even though there was no clinical or radiological suspicion of it.

Charcot deformity and osteomyelitis

Charcot deformity of the foot in diabetes (see also Chapter 7) is relatively common. As the deformity is often associated with intractable secondary neuropathic ulceration (Figure 5.22), there is a very real risk that the deformed bone may become secondarily infected.

Once that occurs, it may prove impossible to eradicate the infection and progressive destruction of the foot will result. However, it is not easy to define secondary infection at an early stage because the clinical and radiological signs of Charcot deformity and of osteomyelitis may be identical. MRI may be diagnostic, but scanning with labelled leucocytes is the most helpful investigation since the false positive rate with uninfected Charcot deformity is very low. Biopsy to establish the presence or otherwise of infection, when the skin is intact, is contraindicated.

Not only does infection commonly complicate secondary infection of an ulcer overlying Charcot deformity, but infection of previously normal tarsal bones may produce collapse and deformity which is itself indistinguishable from a Charcot foot. Secondary infection of a heel ulcer led to progressive destruction of the tarsal bones in the case illustrated in Figure 5.23(a)–(d). Curiously, this woman developed an identical complication of a heel ulcer on the other foot two years later (Figure 5.23(e)–(h)).

Management of osteomyelitis

The orthodox approach to the management of infected bone is to remove it, and limited amputation of an osteomyelitic digit would be recommended by many authorities as the treatment of choice. However, others feel that conservative management should be attempted first and that surgery should be reserved for cases which fail. A number of antibiotic preparations (e.g. co-amoxiclav, clindamycin) have an excellent spectrum of activity against the most likely infecting organisms and are, moreover, well absorbed from the gut and have good bone penetration. Clindamycin and quinolone preparations such as ciprofloxacin and ofloxacin are also concentrated in macrophages, which ensures maximal accumulation at sites of inflammation. Our experience has been that the majority of cases heal completely in response to such conservative management – even when these antibiotics are given orally – and may eliminate the need for admission to hospital. We recommend, however, that such treatment should be continued for not less than 2 months.

Whether osteomyelitis is treated conservatively or surgically, there is always residual deformity. The

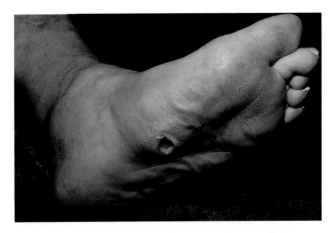

Figure 5.22 The Charcot deformity leads to medial bulging of the tarsal bones, causing increased pressure on the inside of the foot which may ulcerate. When this becomes secondarily infected, it can be impossible to eradicate from the deformed bones beneath.

disorganized bones heal with fusion and shortening (Figure 5.24).

This deformity can lead to new ulcers forming in the future – because of the abnormal distribution of pressure under the deformed foot (Figures 5.25 and 5.26). Fitted footwear is therefore essential.

MICROBIOLOGY

There have been many studies of the organisms likely to be involved in infection of diabetic foot ulcers, and a number of simple conclusions can be drawn.

1. Simple cellulitis is likely to be caused by streptococci and other Gram-positive aerobic bacteria.
2. Subacute and chronic cellulitis is likely to be caused by Gram-positive cocci as well as anaerobes.
3. The infecting organisms in osteomyelitis are usually *S. aureus* and anaerobes.
4. The more ischaemic the foot, and the more necrotic the lesion, the more likely are enterococci and Gram-negative bacilli to be isolated – together with staphylococci, other streptococci and anaerobes.
5. Smell and fever usually indicate anaerobic infection.
6. Gas in the tissue usually indicates anaerobes or Gram-negative bacilli.

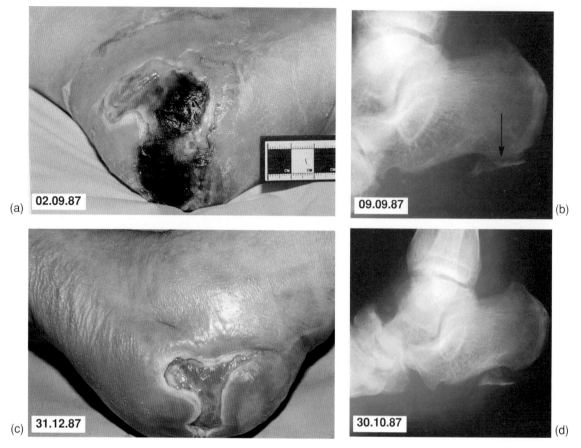

(a) 02.09.87   (b) 09.09.87

(c) 31.12.87   (d) 30.10.87

Figure 5.23(a) This ulcer started when the patient scalded her heel on a hot water bottle. **(b)** An X-ray taken a few days later shows involvement of bone with detachment of the calcaneal spur (arrowed). This appearance is seen in Charcot osteoarthropathy but the presence of an overlying ulcer in this case suggests that it may be the result of osteomyelitis. **(c)** The heel ulcer is healing well after 4 months of regular dressings and treatment with systemic antibiotics. **(d)** The involvement of the calcaneum has been complicated by collapse of the talus and navicular – which could be partly the result of either bone infection or neuropathic osteoarthropathy. If both processes occur at the same time it can be impossible to determine which is clinically more important.

Figure 5.24(a) Osteomyelitis of the hallux with overlying necrotic scab, which was treated conservatively as an outpatient, without admission to hospital. **(b)** The lesion healed well although the toe was typically left shortened and deformed. This would lead to secondary neuropathic ulceration on the tips of the other toes unless fitted shoes were provided.

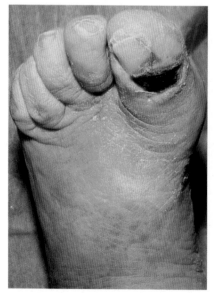
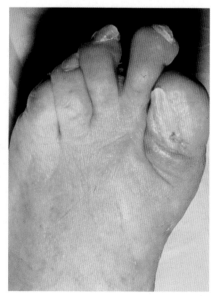

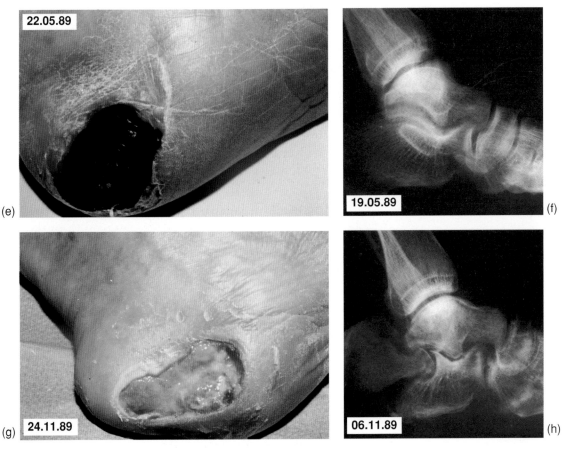

(e) 22.05.89

(f) 19.05.89

(g) 24.11.89

(h) 06.11.89

Figure 5.23(e) This shows the other foot of the woman illustrated in **(a)–(d)**. Just over a year after the lesion on her right foot healed, she burned her left heel on a bath tap – and a nearly identical sequence of events followed. **(f)** At the time of the accident shown in **(e)** the bone texture does not look entirely normal, but there is no overt destruction.

(g) After 6 months of patient nursing care the ulcer shows signs of healing, but it is obvious that the heel itself has changed shape. **(h)** X-ray shows that the calcaneum has disintegrated. The patient died soon after this, of intractable congestive cardiac failure complicating ischaemic heart disease.

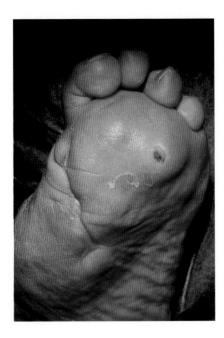

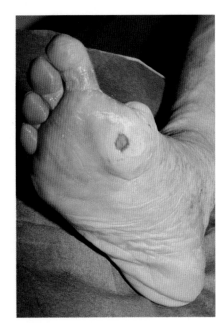

Figure 5.25 (left) Previous surgery for osteomyelitis of the hallux has been complicated by the development of secondary neuropathic ulceration over the third metatarsal head. Such ulcers should not occur if the patient is supplied with appropriate footwear after the operation.

Figure 5.26 (right) This woman also had her osteomyelitis treated by amputation of the hallux. No attention was paid to the provision of surgical shoes to offset the effects of the abnormal weight distribution caused by the surgery, and she too developed a secondary neuropathic ulcer.

Identification

The nature of the infecting organism is identified by culture of material taken from the wound. For most clinical purposes this is done by superficial swabbing of the wound. Note that the swab should be dipped into sterile saline before the sample is taken – especially if the ulcer is relatively dry (Figure 5.27).

In order to obtain the most useful information, material should be obtained by firm probing of the swab tip into the deepest parts of the wound (Figure 5.28).

The swab should then be placed immediately into transport medium and taken to the laboratory as quickly as possible. Exudate can be aspirated into

Figure 5.31 (opposite) A guide to the expected sensitivity of different microorganisms to antibiotic preparations in common use (reproduced from Finch, R.G. (1992) Antibacterial chemotherapy. *Medicine International*, **104**: 4375, by kind permission of The Medicine Group (Journals) Ltd).

a 1 ml syringe for transport to the laboratory (Figure 5.29).

The collection of material for culture, and determination of sensitivity is essential for the proper choice of antibiotic. It is especially important for the exclusion of methicillin-resistant *S. aureus* and *Pseudomonas aeruginosa* – which require special

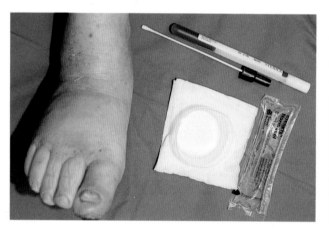

Figure 5.27 Swabs should be moistened with sterile saline before being used. When material has been collected, the swab should be sent to the laboratory as quickly as possible, using a transport medium.

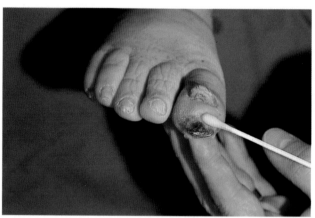

Figure 5.28 Moistened swabs should be pressed into the deepest parts of the wound.

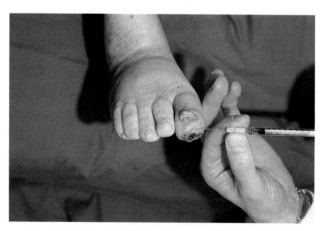

Figure 5.29 Material for culture can be aspirated into a syringe.

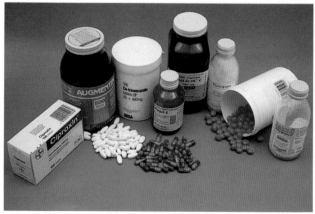

Figure 5.30 A selection of antibiotic preparations which may be used in the management of infection in the diabetic foot.

Sensitivity of selected bacteria to common antibacterial agents

	Staphylococcus aureus (penicillin sensitive)	*Staph aureus* (penicillin resistant)	*Streptococcus pyogenes*[1] and *Strep. pneumoniae*	*Enterococcus faecalis*	*Neisseria gonorrhoeae*	*N. meningitidis*	*Haemophilus influenzae*	*Escherichia coli*	*Klebsiella* spp.	*Proteus mirabilis*	*Serratia* spp.	*Pseudomonas aeruginosa*	*Bacteroides fragilis*	Other *Bacteroides* spp./other anaerobes
Penicillin V/G	Sensitive	Resistant	Some strains resistant	Some strains resistant	Some strains resistant	Sensitive	Some strains resistant	Resistant	Resistant	Resistant	Resistant	Resistant	Resistant	Sensitive
Ampicillin/amoxycillin	Sensitive	Resistant	Some strains resistant	Sensitive	Some strains resistant	Sensitive	Some strains resistant	Some strains resistant	Resistant	Sensitive	Resistant	Resistant	Resistant	Sensitive
Co-amoxiclav	Sensitive	Sensitive	Some strains resistant	Sensitive	Sensitive	Sensitive but not appropriate therapy	Sensitive	Sensitive	Sensitive	Sensitive	Resistant	Resistant	Sensitive	Sensitive
Methicillin/cloxacillin/ flucloxacillin	Sensitive	Sensitive	Some strains resistant	Resistant	Sensitive but not appropriate therapy	Sensitive but not appropriate therapy	Resistant	Resistant	Resistant	Resistant	Resistant	Resistant	Resistant	Resistant
Carbenicillin/ticarcillin	Sensitive but not appropriate therapy	Resistant	Sensitive but not appropriate therapy	Resistant	Sensitive but not appropriate therapy	Sensitive but not appropriate therapy	Sensitive but not appropriate therapy	Some strains resistant	Some strains resistant	Sensitive	Some strains resistant	Some strains resistant	Some strains resistant	Some strains resistant
Cefamandole/cefuroxime	Sensitive	Sensitive	Sensitive	Resistant	Sensitive but not appropriate therapy	Sensitive but not appropriate therapy	Sensitive	Sensitive	Sensitive	Sensitive	Resistant	Resistant	Some strains resistant	Sensitive
Cefoxitin	Sensitive	Sensitive	Sensitive	Resistant	Sensitive but not appropriate therapy	Sensitive but not appropriate therapy	Sensitive	Sensitive	Sensitive	Sensitive	Some strains resistant	Resistant	Sensitive	Sensitive
Cefotaxime	Sensitive	Sensitive	Sensitive	Resistant	Sensitive	Sensitive	Sensitive	Sensitive	Sensitive	Sensitive	Sensitive	Some strains resistant	Some strains resistant	Some strains resistant
Ceftazidime	Sensitive	Sensitive	Sensitive	Resistant	Sensitive	Sensitive	Sensitive	Sensitive	Sensitive	Sensitive	Sensitive	Sensitive	Resistant	Some strains resistant
Aztreonam	Resistant	Resistant	Resistant	Resistant	Sensitive	Sensitive	Sensitive	Sensitive	Sensitive	Sensitive	Sensitive	Sensitive	Resistant	Resistant
Erythromycin	Some strains resistant	Some strains resistant	Some strains resistant	Resistant	Sensitive	Sensitive but not appropriate therapy	Some strains resistant	Resistant	Resistant	Resistant	Resistant	Resistant	Some strains resistant	Sensitive
Clindamycin	Sensitive	Sensitive	Sensitive	Resistant	Resistant	Resistant	Resistant	Resistant	Resistant	Resistant	Resistant	Resistant	Sensitive	Sensitive
Tetracyclines	Some strains resistant	Some strains resistant	Some strains resistant	Resistant	Sensitive	Sensitive but not appropriate therapy	Sensitive	Sensitive	Some strains resistant	Some strains resistant	Resistant	Resistant	Some strains resistant	Sensitive
Chloramphenicol	Sensitive but not appropriate therapy	Sensitive but not appropriate therapy	Sensitive	Sensitive	Sensitive but not appropriate therapy	Sensitive	Sensitive	Sensitive	Sensitive	Sensitive	Sensitive	Resistant	Sensitive	Sensitive
Mecillinam	Resistant	Resistant	Sensitive	Resistant	Resistant	Resistant	Resistant	Sensitive	Sensitive	Sensitive	Sensitive	Resistant	Resistant	Sensitive
Gentamicin/tobramycin/ netilmicin/amikacin	Sensitive	Sensitive	Resistant	Resistant	Sensitive but not appropriate therapy	Sensitive but not appropriate therapy	Sensitive but not appropriate therapy	Sensitive	Sensitive	Sensitive	Sensitive	Sensitive	Resistant	Resistant
Sulphonamides	Sensitive	Sensitive	Some strains resistant	Some strains resistant	Some strains resistant	Some strains resistant	Some strains resistant	Some strains resistant	Resistant	Some strains resistant	Resistant	Resistant	Resistant	Resistant
Co-trimoxazole	Sensitive	Sensitive	Sensitive	Sensitive	Sensitive	Sensitive	Sensitive	Sensitive	Sensitive	Sensitive	Resistant	Resistant	Resistant	Resistant
Trimethoprim	Sensitive	Sensitive	Sensitive	Sensitive	Resistant	Resistant	Sensitive	Some strains resistant	Some strains resistant	Some strains resistant	Some strains resistant	Resistant	Resistant	Resistant
Ciprofloxacin	Sensitive	Sensitive	Sensitive	Sensitive	Sensitive	Sensitive	Sensitive	Sensitive	Sensitive	Sensitive	Sensitive	Sensitive	Resistant	Resistant

Sensitive — Sensitive but not appropriate therapy

Resistant — Some strains resistant

[1] *Strep. pyogenes* remains sensitive to penicillins.

approaches to management. It should be noted, however, that swabs are only of value if they are taken carefully and sent rapidly to the laboratory, in an appropriate transport medium. Without such attention to detail, the only organisms isolated will be those that are most robust, usually *S. aureus*.

Management of infection

Infection is responsible for delayed healing of wounds, and can contribute to progressive devital-ization of tissue. It can also precipitate the development of gangrene, as described above. It is important, therefore, for it to be recognized early and treated aggressively. Appropriate antibiotics should be used early (without waiting for the swab result).

GENERAL MEASURES

1. The patient should rest the foot as much as possible (at least in the short term). If the lesion persists for more than a week or so, it becomes impractical for a person to rest completely and advice has to be tailored accordingly.
2. Antibiotics should be administered orally. In cases of obviously severe sepsis, the patient should be referred urgently to a specialist unit for consideration of admission and parenteral therapy.
3. General hygiene and cleansing of the wound: although the infection will be cleared only with appropriate systemic antibiotics and the choice of cleansing agent and dressing is unlikely to modify the rate of healing, it is important to clean and dress the wound at least daily. The objectives are twofold: first, to prevent superadded infection by keeping the surface as clean as possible and second, to make sure that the lesion is checked regularly for signs of deterioration. Many doctors and nurses tell patients not to get the foot wet or to have a bath while the ulcer persists. Given that the average healing time of ulcers is of the order of 3 months, this imposes an unnecessary and unhealthy restriction on the patient (see Figure 10.16). There is no evidence to suggest that an ulcer is made worse by being put in the bath; the chances are that it is helped.

CHOICE OF ANTIBIOTIC

The choice of antibiotic preparations is large (Figure 5.30), but selection depends on the nature of the likely infecting organism, the type and severity of the infection and patient factors such as drug sensitivity. The spectrum of commonly used oral and intravenous antibiotics and their activity against different organisms, is shown in Figure 5.31.

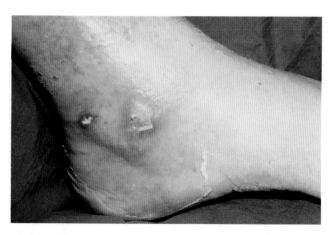

Figure 5.32 Uncomplicated soft tissue infection should respond to a penicillin, a cephalosporin or erythromycin. The presence of pus, as here, suggests involvement with *S. aureus* and in such cases it is best to add agents with particular activity against it, such as flucloxacillin, fusidic acid, clindamycin or co-amoxiclav.

Table 5.1 Suitable preparations for the management of uncomplicated cellulitis

Oral	Intravenous
Amoxycillin	Ampicillin, benzyl penicillin, cefuroxime
Erythromycin	

Uncomplicated cellulitis

In uncomplicated soft tissue infection (Figure 5.32 and Table 5.1), a penicillin preparation (e.g. amoxycillin or pivampicillin) should be sufficient. A cephalosporin or macrolide (erythromycin) could be used in those who are penicillin-sensitive.

Severe soft tissue infection

When there is more extensive devitalized tissue, there is more likely to be a mixed spectrum of organisms and a broad-spectrum regimen must be chosen (Figure 5.33 and Table 5.2).

Broad-spectrum cover can be provided orally with co-amoxiclav, or a combination of a quinolone (e.g. ofloxacin) and metronidazole. A suitable intravenous regimen for those who are not penicillin-sensitive is ampicillin and gentamicin, in combination with oral or rectal metronidazole.

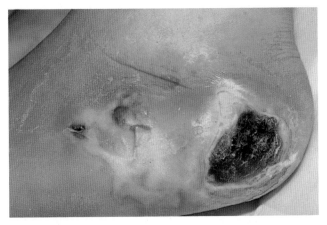

Figure 5.33 More extensive infection of soft tissues requires a broad-spectrum regimen, and treatment should be parenteral in the first instance. The presence of extensive devitalized tissue is a very poor prognostic sign – even though the leg may occasionally be saved with a combination of effective antibiotic therapy and appropriate surgery (see cover illustration).

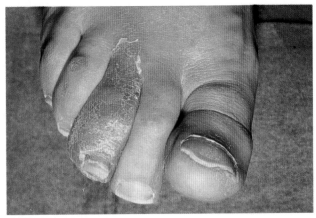

Figure 5.34 Typical appearance of osteomyelitis affecting the third toe. It should respond well to conservative therapy, although the antibiotics chosen should be active against both anaerobes and Gram-positive aerobic cocci and need to be given for at least 2 months.

Table 5.2 Suitable preparations for treatment of likely mixed infection

Oral	Intravenous

Co-amoxiclav**
 Ofloxacin*
	Ampicillin and gentamicin*
	 Cefotaxime*
	 More expensive regimens:
	    Ceftazidime
	    Imipenem

* combined with oral or rectal metronidazole
** can be used parenterally as well

Table 5.3 Suitable preparations for the conservative management of osteomyelitis

Oral**	Intravenous
Clindamycin Co-amoxiclav Flucloxacillin and fusidate* Ofloxacin*	Ampicillin and gentamicin* Cefotaxime*

* with oral or rectal metronidazole
** can be used parenterally as well

Osteomyelitis

Osteomyelitis (Figure 5.34) can usually be managed conservatively.

Oral regimens are often adequate but must be continued for at least 2 months. Both clindamycin and co-amoxiclav give the necessary cover against Gram-positive cocci and anaerobes (Table 5.3). Intravenous therapy is indicated in more severe cases, and those who do not respond should have the affected bone excised.

6 Vasculopathy

INTRODUCTION

The role of the vascular system is to deliver oxygen and nutrients to cells. When the blood supply is impaired, the integrity of the skin and subcutaneous tissue of the foot is reduced: they are more liable to ulcerate in response to minor injury, and less likely to heal once broken. If bacteria enter through the break in the skin and cause secondary infection, the situation worsens. The body is unable to eliminate the infection from ischaemic tissue quickly because the inflammatory response is reduced, with defective delivery of neutrophils, monocytes and specific anti-bodies. The bacteria compete with normal cells for oxygen and nutrients and may also worsen the delivery of blood to the area by causing clotting of smaller vessels. Underlying ischaemia is the most important single factor leading to delay of ulcer healing and, potentially, to loss of the limb.

NORMAL INFLAMMATORY PROCESS

When cells are damaged, they release a series of cytokines and locally active factors that stimulate the inflammatory process (Figure 6.1).

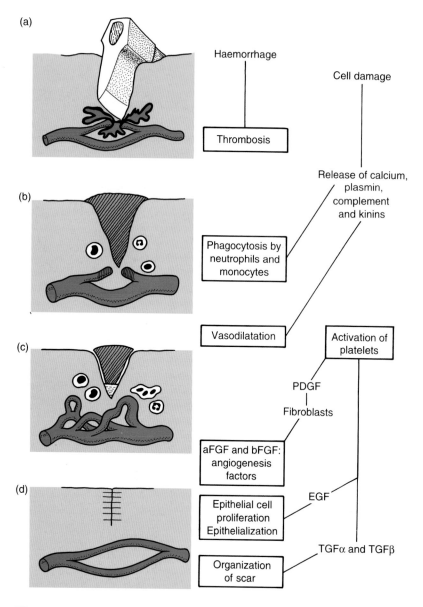

Figure 6.1 Healing after penetrating injury.

(a) Wounding: Haemorrhage and cell damage result in the release of a variety of cytokines. These then result in the arrest of haemorrhage by thrombosis, and the start of the repair process.

(b) Damage limitation: Neutrophils and monocytes accumulate in the area, and remove damaged and foreign material. Vasodilatation of arterioles and venules brings increased blood to the site. The role of platelets appears to be central to the healing process. Not only are they the key to the thrombotic cascade, but they also initiate the healing process by the release of a variety of growth factors (GFs).

(c) Damage repair: Platelet-derived growth factors (PDGF) lead to the proliferation of fibroblasts and other connective tissue. Fibroblasts release acidic and basic fibroblast growth factors (aFGF and bFGF) which appear to be the main stimuli to the formation of new blood vessels.

(d) Healing: The secretion by platelets of epidermal growth factor (EGF) and transforming growth factors (TGFα and TGFβ) helps complete wound healing.

The key features of the process are:

1. thrombosis to stop haemorrhage;
2. mobilization of neutrophils and macrophages to eliminate foreign material, including bacteria;
3. vasodilatation and new vessel formation to cope with the increased needs of cells dividing rapidly to heal the injury;
4. epithelialization;
5. organization of scar tissue.

The subject is also discussed in Chapter 10.

Thrombosis

There is no impairment of thrombosis in diabetes. Indeed, there is some suggestion of an increased tendency to clotting in small blood vessels. Thus haemorrhage is arrested normally, but there is inappropriate thrombosis in the small vessels which surround the area and this results in a reduced, rather than an increased supply of blood to the damaged tissues. Such inappropriate thrombosis is especially likely in small arteries already narrowed by atheroma and capillaries made rigid by thickening of the basement membrane (see below).

Mobilization of neutrophils and monocytes

The ability of white blood cells to migrate into areas of inflammation and to ingest microorganisms is reduced in diabetes. At least, phagocytosis and resistance to infection is reduced in diabetics with a high blood sugar; it is normal in those who are normoglycaemic.

Vasodilatation and new vessel formation

The ability of small vessels to dilate may be diminished by small vessel disease (see below).

Epithelialization and organization

The proliferation of new vessels, connective tissue and epidermis requires a complex interaction between growth factors released locally. Only some of these are illustrated in Figure 6.1; the subject is poorly understood.

MACROVASCULAR DISEASE

The term 'macrovascular disease' refers to narrowing of larger arteries by atherosclerosis (Figure 6.2). It is more common in people with diabetes.

Atherosclerosis

The development of atherosclerosis is the result partly of metabolic defects and partly of physical ones. The accumulation of lipids in the cell wall is caused by fat-filled monocytes passing through the endothelium from the circulation (Figure 6.3).

This process is exaggerated when serum lipid concentrations are high, and is virtually unknown if the cholesterol is less than 4 mmol/l. However, other processes are involved, many of which are mediated by changes in activity of local growth factors, including platelet-derived growth factor (PDGF) and insulin-like growth factor 1 (IGF_1). These lead to smooth muscle proliferation, loss of elastin, fibrosis

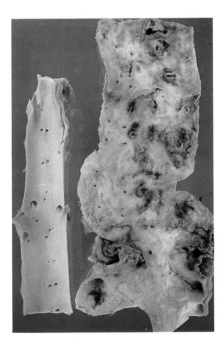

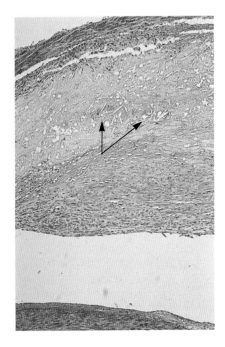

Figure 6.2 (left) The appearance of the normal aorta at post-mortem (left) contrasts with the gross distortion resulting from severe atherosclerosis. Numerous atheromatous plaques are visible, which narrow the lumen, act as a base for thrombus formation and are liable to rupture and embolize.

Figure 6.3 (right) A plaque of atheroma lies within the lumen of a medium-sized artery. Proliferation of smooth muscle and fibrous tissue is clearly visible as are fatty deposits and 'cholesterol clefts' (arrowed).

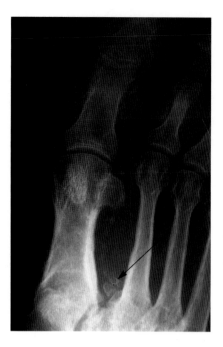

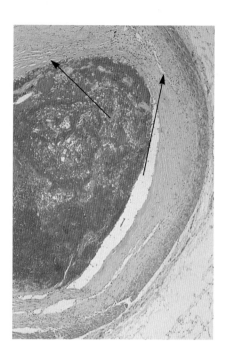

Figure 6.4 (left) The media of vessels affected by atherosclerosis often becomes calcified, and this may be visible on plain X-ray (arrowed).

Figure 6.5 (right) Once atherosclerosis affects the intima by distension, or by rupturing through it, it acts as a focus for thrombosis – which may occlude the vessel altogether. This figure shows the fibrous proliferation and fatty deposits of the atherosclerosis lying within the vessel wall (arrowed), as well as the large central plug of thrombus.

and calcification. The calcification of the arteries in the foot can be visible on plain X-ray (Figure 6.4).

The swollen fibro-fatty mass of atheroma then ulcerates through the intima, when one of three things may happen.

1. It may cause chronic, slowly progressive obstruction to the flow of blood.
2. Secondary thrombosis may further worsen the blood flow, sometimes acutely (Figure 6.5).
3. Either atheroma or secondary thrombus may detach and cause embolic ischaemia of distal tissues.
   <<Fig. 6.5 here>>

Hypertension and hyperlipidaemia

A number of factors are associated with increased risk of atherosclerosis (Table 6.1).
<<Table 6.1 here>>

Attempts should be made to reduce high blood pressure and gross hyperlipidaemia if possible, but it remains to be established whether the late (and many of these people are elderly) reduction of mild to moderate hyperlipidaemia is of any value. Any benefit has to be offset against the possibility that attempts at reduction might be either physically or psychologically harmful.

Smoking

The single intervention which helps even in those with established severe disease is the cessation of smoking. Smoking both exacerbates the formation of atherosclerosis (partly by the irritant effect of carbon monoxide) and increases the likelihood of secondary thrombosis. The group of younger insulin-dependent

Table 6.1 Risk factors for the development of atherosclerosis

Metabolic
　Hyperglycaemia
　Hypercholesterolaemia
　Hypertriglyceridaemia
　Reduced HDL cholesterol
　Increased oxidative stress (free radicals)
　Hypercoagulability
　Hyperinsulinaemia

Physical
　Hypertension

Constitutional
　Gender
　Familial predisposition
　Age
　Obesity

Social
　Smoking

diabetics who are particularly at risk of foot problems is that of men who smoke.

Oral contraceptives and hormone replacement therapy

The proper use of oral contraceptives in diabetes has not been clearly established. Although many recommend the use of progesterone-only pills, there is little conclusive evidence of increased risk of vascular disease in diabetics who use 30 μg combined preparations. The choice of a preparation with a less androgenic progestogen, such as desogestrel, may be preferable, as may the 20 μg equivalent. Hormone replacement therapy (HRT) is not contraindicated in diabetes. Indeed, the increase in cardiovascular risk in women with diabetes is a relatively strong indication for recommending HRT.

MICROVASCULAR DISEASE

Not only is diabetes associated with an increased tendency to atherosclerosis leading to reduction in delivery of blood to the small arteries and arterioles, but there is also defective transfer of oxygen and nutrients across the capillary walls as a result of microvascular disease (Figure 6.6).

Microvascular disease takes three forms:

1. thickening of the capillary basement membrane leading to impairment of the transfer of nutrients across the vessel wall (Figure 6.7);

2. thrombosis of the capillaries – probably because they are made less elastic by the thickened basement membrane and red blood cells are unable to pass through them;

3. abnormal shunting of blood as a result of disease of vasomotor nerves (Figure 6.8). Thus, it may not be possible for the body to divert blood efficiently to the part where it is needed, i.e. in order to hasten ulcer healing.

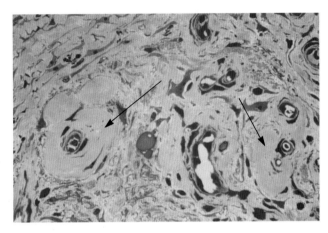

Figure 6.7 Gross thickening of the basement membrane which surrounds the endothelial cells of the capillaries in diabetes (arrowed). This limits the transfer of nutrients across the vessel wall and also makes the vessel more rigid and hence more liable to clot.

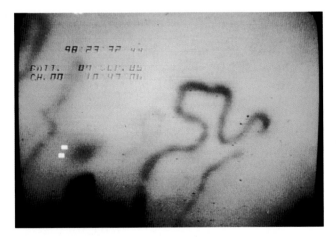

Figure 6.6 It is now possible to study the vascular dynamics of small blood vessels *in vivo*. Nail fold capillaries such as that shown can be directly cannulated and assessment can be made of their luminal pressure and flow in response to different stimuli.

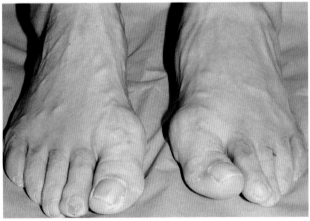

Figure 6.8 Autonomic neuropathy affecting the vasomotor nerves in the foot leads to arteriovenous shunting. The veins are distended and the foot is warm. Both the pressure and the oxygen content of the veins is increased. The dorsalis pedis pulse may be easily felt, and even exaggerated, but the skin and peripheral tissues can be ischaemic because they are bypassed.

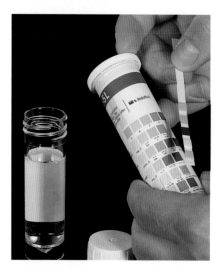

Figure 6.9 The presence of proteinuria is a poor prognostic sign in diabetes: it reflects disease of the capillaries of the renal glomeruli and is nearly always associated with vascular disease elsewhere. The majority have retinopathy and hypertension; 30% will have a myocardial infarction within 6 years of the onset of proteinuria.

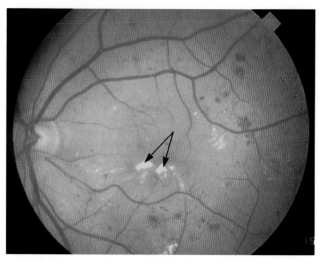

Figure 6.10 Microvascular disease in the eye – microvascular aneurysms and haemorrhage, associated with hard exudates (arrowed). Patients with diabetic foot ulcers should have their eyes examined regularly, through dilated pupils. Of patients whose diabetes is only discovered when they present with a foot ulcer, 40% will have retinopathy at the time of presentation.

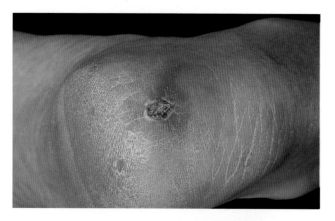

Figure 6.11 Cracks tend to be worst around the heel. They may be cracks or more rounded infarcts, as shown here. They are the result of skin ischaemia and can be very painful.

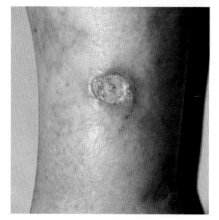

Figure 6.12 Lesions can appear spontaneously on the shins as a result of medium-to-small vessel occlusion. They may be very slow to heal – despite the presence of healthy-looking granulation tissue. They can also be very painful.

People with microvascular disease of the foot may well have signs of microvascular disease elsewhere, e.g. nephropathy and retinopathy. All should have their urine examined for protein (Figure 6.9) and their fundi examined for retinopathy through dilated pupils (Figure 6.10).

IDENTIFICATION OF ISCHAEMIA IN THE DIABETIC FOOT

Acute obstruction of the large arteries of the leg by thrombus or embolus results in a cold, white, painful leg which is a surgical emergency. It is not, however, a particular feature of diabetes and is beyond the scope of this book. More chronic obstruction of the large arteries of the leg results in intermittent claudication. However, the vast majority of ischaemic lesions of the foot in diabetes are painless. There are only a few types that typically present with pain: infarcts or cracks on the heels (Figure 6.11), infarcts on the back of the shin (Figure 6.12) and some chronic ulcers over bony prominences (often called 'neuroischaemic ulcers') which have become secondarily infected (see Figure 5.13).

Paradoxically, the symptom of having cold feet does not always indicate poor circulation: it can indicate peripheral neuropathy rather than peripheral vascular disease (see Chapter 7).

Signs of chronic ischaemia

The signs of ischaemia are several. The skin is thin, red, dry and shiny (Figure 6.13). The nails tend to be slow-growing, and are often short and dystrophic (Figure 6.14). There may be multiple superficial scabs over the tips of the toes and the knuckles – indicating damage at points of normal, minor trauma which is slow to heal (Figure 6.15).

Critical reduction in arterial blood flow is demonstrated by Buerger's test – in which the affected limb is pale when elevated, but goes dark purple when it hangs over the side of the bed (Figure 6.16). Similarly, it is possible to show delayed capillary return in the elevated leg (blanching in response to pressure from the thumb). The pulses of the foot will be impalpable (Figure 6.17).

Typical lesions of the ischaemic foot

NEUROISCHAEMIC ULCERS

These include those superficial, not obviously infected sores which are seen over the malleoli and over the medial aspect of the first metatarsophalangeal joint ('neuroischaemic' ulcers) (Figure 6.18). Similar ulcers occur between the toes ('kissing' ulcers) (Figure 6.19).

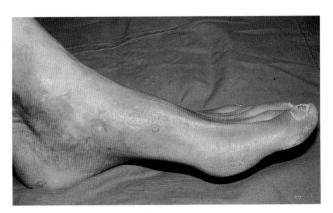

Figure 6.13 The ischaemic foot has thin, red, shiny skin. It also tends to be dry from loss of sweating, and hairless.

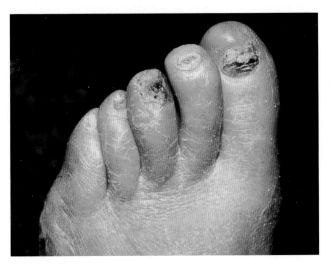

Figure 6.14 Dry, flaking skin in the ischaemic foot, together with dystrophic nails (discoloured by application of povidone-iodine).

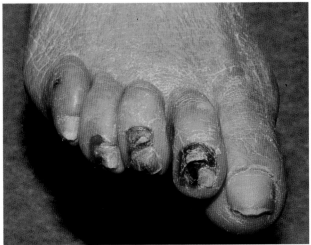

Figure 6.15 The skin of an ischaemic foot is unable to withstand the pressure and shearing forces of shoes and normal walking. It breaks down, leaving scabs, typically over the knuckles of the toes.

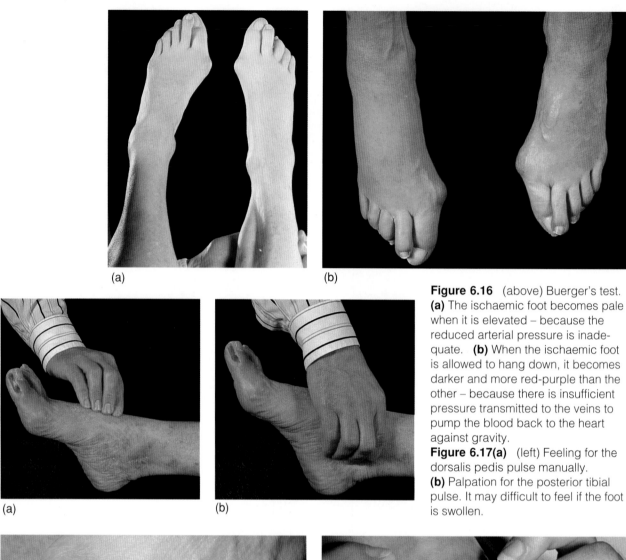

(a) (b)

(a) (b)

Figure 6.16 (above) Buerger's test.
(a) The ischaemic foot becomes pale when it is elevated – because the reduced arterial pressure is inadequate. **(b)** When the ischaemic foot is allowed to hang down, it becomes darker and more red-purple than the other – because there is insufficient pressure transmitted to the veins to pump the blood back to the heart against gravity.

Figure 6.17(a) (left) Feeling for the dorsalis pedis pulse manually.
(b) Palpation for the posterior tibial pulse. It may difficult to feel if the foot is swollen.

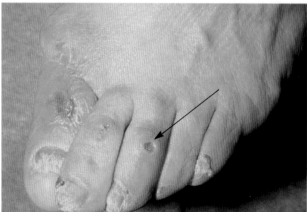

Figure 6.18 Most ischaemic feet are also neuropathic, because the nerves themselves are ischaemic. Thus the person may develop an ulcer at a site of increased pressure, caused for example by ill-fitting footwear (arrowed), and be unaware of it because of reduced sensation. The ulcer tends to be superficial and, because the skin is short of nutrients, there is no gross build-up of callus as seen in the classical 'neuropathic' type.

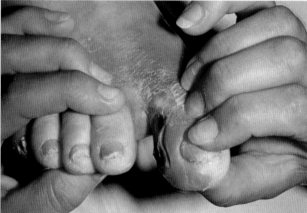

Figure 6.19 Neuroischaemic ulceration between the toes occurs as a result of lateral pressure and vertical shearing forces. These ulcers are slow to heal and may become secondarily infected, as shown here by the spread of erythema into the forefoot.

ULCERS OF THE HEEL

Heel ulcers nearly always indicate ischaemia: both the large painless ulcers resulting (usually) from immobilization (Figure 6.20), as well as small painful ones (Figure 6.21). Ischaemic infarcts result from occlusion of a small end-artery and are also exquisitely painful. They tend to occur on the side of the heel and the back of the shin (Figure 6.12).

BLISTERS

Blisters may also occur in the ischaemic foot – often in response to minimal trauma (Figure 6.22). They are seen most commonly in people with low cardiac output complicating chronic congestive cardiac failure, but can occur also in those with severe autonomic neuropathy. They occur because ischaemia of the more superficial layers of the skin results in loss of the anchoring fibrils and liability to separation when subjected to minor shearing forces.

UNHEALING ULCERS

The ischaemia of tissues may be evident from the chronic persistence of superficial, granulating but unhealing ulcers on the shin. The epidermis is unable to complete the healing process by epithelialization: sometimes the ulcers close over at one end, only to extend at the other (Figure 6.23). A similar situation is seen in operation wounds which fail to heal by secondary intention when the superficial tissues are ischaemic (Figure 6.24).

INVESTIGATION OF ISCHAEMIA

Examination of peripheral pulses by Doppler

Pulses which are hard to feel may be identified more easily using a Doppler probe to detect systolic pressure. In the non-ischaemic foot, the pressure is similar (±20%) to the level in the brachial artery. Values below 0.8 of the brachial in either the posterior tibial or the dorsalis pedis indicate significant reduction in large vessel flow (Figure 6.25).

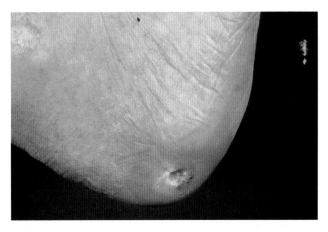

Figure 6.21 This small ulcer started when the patient was in bed after a stroke. It was very painful and persisted until he died 10 years later.

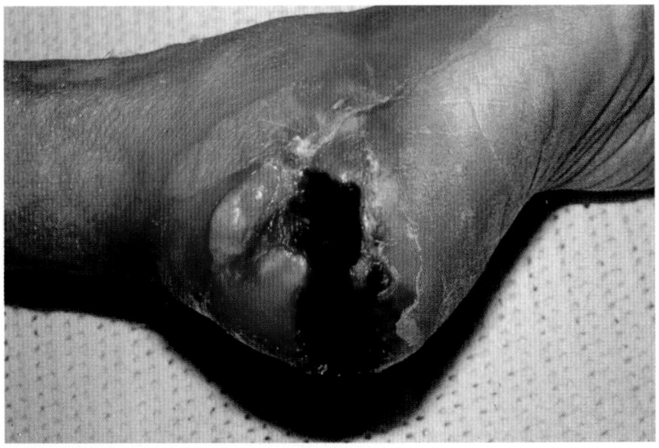

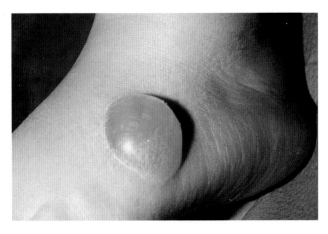

Figure 6.22 Blisters occur when the skin is rendered ischaemic by macrovascular disease, arteriovenous shunting or both. Premature ageing with loss of anchoring fibrils makes the dermoepidermal junction susceptible to minor shearing forces.

Figure 6.20 A large painless ulcer on the heel. The ulcer healed in response to prolonged nursing care, only to break down again and remain unhealed until the patient died.

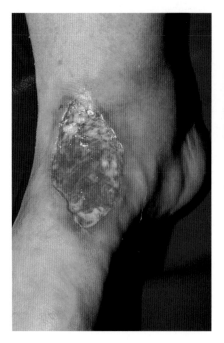

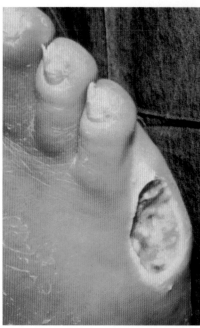

Figure 6.23 (far left) Superficial granulating ulcers of the shin can persist for many months, often healing at one end while extending at the other.

Figure 6.24 (left) Amputation of the gangrenous toe is avoided in the ischaemic foot, if possible, for fear that the wound will not heal. The wound here looks pale and inert and has few signs of active inflammation.

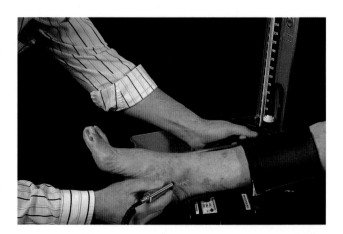

Figure 6.25 A hand-held Doppler probe can be used to detect systolic blood pressure in the posterior tibial and dorsalis pedis pulses. The ratio of the pressure in the foot to that in the brachial artery (ABI, ankle brachial index) should be between 0.8 and 1.2. If the vessels in the calf are very sclerotic, it may be impossible to compress them with the sphygmomanometer cuff, and this may result in an artificially high ABI – even in the presence of severe peripheral vascular disease.

Artefactually high readings are occasionally encountered in atherosclerosis: the blood flow can be very poor but it may be impossible to compress vessels in the calf with the sphygmomanometer cuff if they are heavily calcified.

Toe plethysmography

Toe blood flow can be determined using toe plethysmography, using a mercury–rubber strain gauge.

Transcutaneous oxygen tension

Measurement of transcutaneous oxygen tension TcO_2 is a simple bedside method of determining the degree of oxygenation of the tissues.

Duplex ultrasonography

Duplex ultrasound is a non-invasive technique that can be used to calculate blood flow rate in any of the larger vessels of the leg (Figure 6.26), and is increasingly used in specialist vascular units in place of invasive angiography. Its main value is in determining the patency of short sections of major arteries.

Angiography

The structure, patency and, to some extent, the flow rate in the arteries can be demonstrated by angiography. The objective is to define an obstruction which is amenable either to bypass surgery or to dilatation by angioplasty.

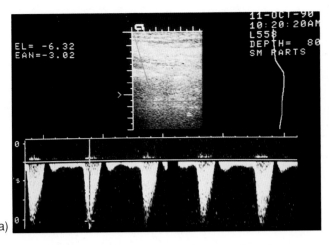

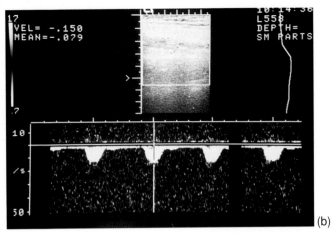

(a)

(b)

Figure 6.26(a) Duplex ultrasound is a non-invasive method that combines measurement of blood velocity with anatomical changes in the blood vessels. The ultrasound picture in **(b)** was taken at the same time as that in **(a)**. It shows a vessel distal to a major stenosis with considerable damping of arterial flow.

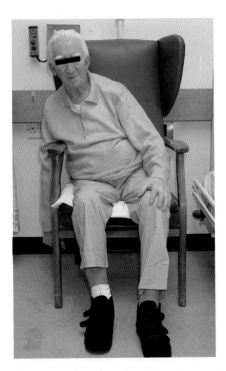

Figure 6.27 Age and pre-existing disease are not necessarily a bar to angiography and arterial surgery. The patient incapacitated by a preceding stroke is less able to cope with the loss of a leg than someone who was previously fit, and every effort should be made to avoid it.

WHEN SHOULD ANGIOGRAPHY BE DONE?

The decision is usually taken only by vascular surgeons, or in specialized units for the management of diabetic foot ulcers. There is no point in considering it in any person who has easily palpable foot pulses because vascular surgery would have nothing to offer in such a case. Similarly, it is not usually considered in people with an easily palpable popliteal pulse because bypass surgery and angioplasty are usually reserved for stenoses above the knee. Nevertheless, treatment of stenoses of smaller vessels is being increasingly undertaken as techniques improve.

Any person should be considered for angiography, irrespective of their overall frailty – provided it is considered that their limb could be saved by intervention and provided they would be able to tolerate the procedure and any subsequent surgery. Even the patient with a foot ulcer who has had a major medical problem such as a stroke should be considered for angiography: s/he will be more incapacitated by amputation than someone without pre-existing disease (Figure 6.27).

Angiography should be considered in any lesion in which there is clinical evidence of significant ischaemia. This includes those presenting with either incipient (Figure 6.28) or established (Figure 6.29) gangrene. It also includes any of the lesions illustrated above (Figures 6.11, 6.12, 6.18–24).

HAVING AN ANGIOGRAM PERFORMED

Angiography is not particularly pleasant for the patient. It involves admission to hospital for at least

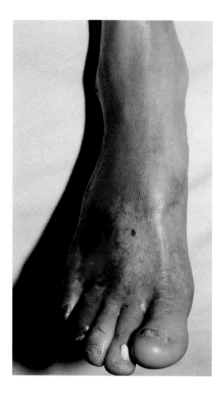

Figure 6.28 (left) The whole foot is ischaemic and the dead skin has sloughed off over the base of the fourth and fifth toes. Unless it is possible to re-establish arterial flow as an emergency, this foot will be lost.

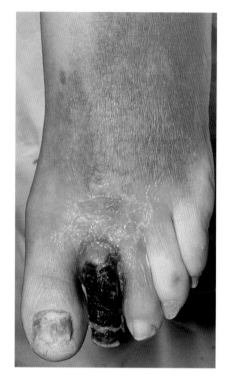

Figure 6.29 (right) Gangrene is the cardinal sign of ischaemia. Gangrene of the single digit like this occurs when paired digital arteries which are already narrowed by atheroma are occluded completely by thrombosis. As often as not, this thrombosis is secondary to spreading soft tissue infection. The signs of resolving infection are apparent in this photograph.

one night. The procedure takes 45 minutes to one hour; it is done under local anaesthesia and is potentially frightening (Figure 6.30). The radio-opaque dye used can hurt as it flows down an ischaemic leg.

The catheter is introduced via a needle inserted in the femoral artery (Figure 6.31).

The catheter tip is then placed either in the lower aorta or in the common iliac arteries and the dye is injected. Conventional radiography produces white on black images (Figure 6.32) although digital subtraction imaging (DSA) is increasingly preferred because of the greater definition of the films (Figure 6.33).

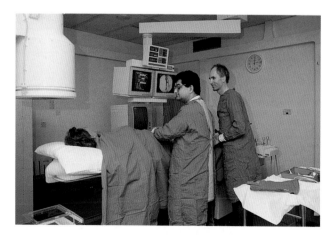

Figure 6.30 Percutaneous angiography is performed under local anaesthetic and is a potentially frightening procedure.

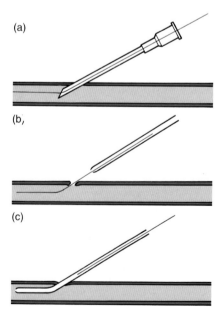

(a)

(b)

(c)

Figure 6.31 The Seldinger technique is used to introduce a flexible plastic cannula into the lower aorta for injection of contrast.

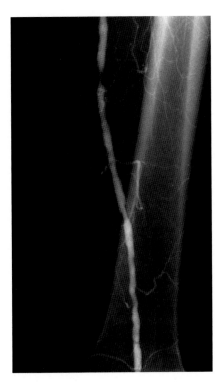

Figure 6.32 (left) Multiple stenoses of the superficial femoral artery demonstrated with conventional contrast techniques.

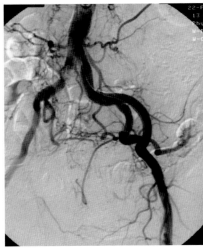

Figure 6.33 (left) Digital subtraction imaging allows greater definition of the vessels.

TREATMENT OF MACROVASCULAR DISEASE

Angioplasty

The technique is very similar to that used in performing an angiogram. The difference is that there is a balloon on the catheter tip. The tip is then introduced into a section of narrowed artery before being distended with normal saline (Figure 6.34). The distended balloon stretches the thrombosed and atheromatous vessel to restore patency. Angioplasty has made an enormous contribution to the management of ischaemic limbs (Figure 6.35).

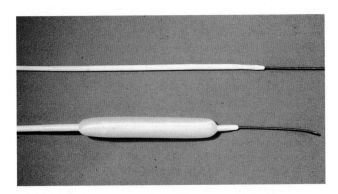

Figure 6.34 Percutaneous intraluminal angioplasty is performed by inserting a catheter with an uninflated balloon (upper). Distension of the balloon with saline stretches the atherosclerotic narrowing of the artery (reproduced by kind permission of Meadox (UK) Ltd).

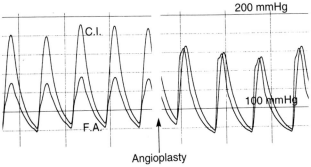

Figure 6.35 This trace superimposes intra-arterial pressures above and below a stenosis in the external iliac artery. In the left half there is a high peak proximal to the block (C.I., common iliac artery) and a lower one distal (F.A., femoral artery). The recordings on the right were made after the narrowing was distended by angioplasty and shows the proximal and distal pressures equalized.

Angioplasty is most suitable for the treatment of short stenoses, preferably in more proximal vessels and ones in which the distal part of the vessel is obviously patent (Figure 6.36). However, progressive advance of the balloon will allow recanalization of blockages several centimetres long (Figure 6.37).

The process of angioplasty can cause quite gross distortion of the architecture of the vessel, with splitting of the intima and media (Figure 6.38). Haemorrhage is a very rare complication, but restenosis by thrombosis is common – especially in longer lesions (Figure 6.39).

Figure 6.36(a) Localized stenoses of the popliteal artery, with some collateral vessel formation. **(b)** The same vessel following angioplasty; the catheter is still in position. Note the roughness of the stretched lumen, with splits and cracks in the intima and media.

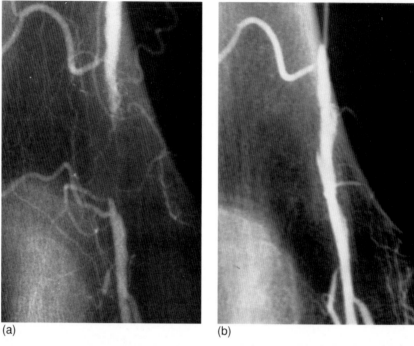

(a)   (b)

Figure 6.37(a) Extensive stenoses of the lower part of the superficial femoral and popliteal arteries. **(b)** Progressive advance of a catheter can be used to distend such long sections of narrowed vessel.

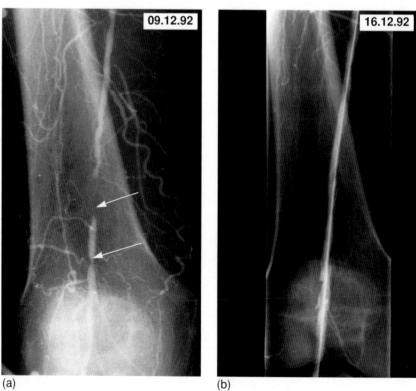

(a)   (b)

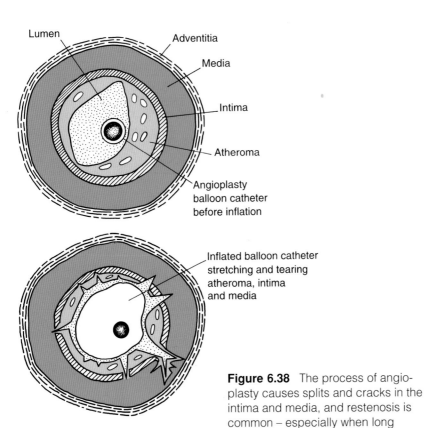

Figure 6.38 The process of angioplasty causes splits and cracks in the intima and media, and restenosis is common – especially when long sections have been treated.

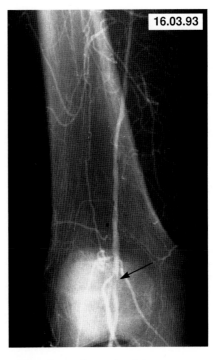

16.03.93

Figure 6.39 Stenosis of the same vessels shown in Figure 6.37 after 3 months. The patient subsequently underwent successful bypass surgery.

A large multicentre study in the USA demonstrated that despite an exponential increase in the numbers of lower limb angioplasties performed in the last 10 years, there has been no reduction in either the numbers of bypass operations undertaken or the number of amputations (Table 6.2).

STENTS

Radiologists and vascular surgeons are starting to explore the use of stents (Figure 6.40) to maintain the patency of previously narrowed vessels.

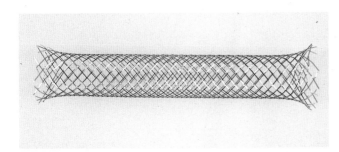

Figure 6.40 Insertion of wire cage stents may maintain the patency of distended vessels.

Table 6.2 The role of angioplasty in limb salvage. Maryland hospitals serve a population of approximately 7 million. Between 1979 and 1989 there was a 400% increase in lower limb angioplasty and a 240% increase in bypass surgery. In the same 11-year period there was no significant change in the rate of lower extremity amputation. The mean age at which lower extremity amputation was performed did not alter either, suggesting that any overall delaying effect of revascularization procedures was not marked. The combined costs of angioplasty and bypass surgery in 1989 were estimated at $30.5 million (data of Tunis SR *et al.* (1991) New England Journal of Medicine, **325**: 556–562).

	Angioplasty	Bypass surgery	Lower extremity amputation
1979	36	1841	1775
1989	1450	4431	2272

Thrombolysis

Thrombus which has formed recently (i.e. within 2–3 weeks) may be dissolved by the intra-arterial instillation of thrombolytic drugs such as streptokinase (Figure 6.41).

Although of potential value, its place in the management of ischaemia in diabetes is limited because most stenoses are chronic. There is also a possibility that a diabetic who has received streptokinase following myocardial infarction may have developed antibodies to it. Streptokinase is also the active ingredient in the desloughing agent Varidase; the antibody status of those treated with this application (see Chapter 10) has not been investigated.

Arterial surgery

Bypass surgery is usually reserved for more extensive lesions above the knee, i.e. long stenoses of the iliac and/or superficial femoral arteries. However, surgery below the knee is being performed with increasing frequency using grafts extending to the posterior tibial artery, or to anterior tibial/dorsalis pedis. The main requirement for such a procedure is the presence of a patent distal vessel to which the graft can be attached (Figure 6.42). The different types of operation are illustrated in Figure 6.43.

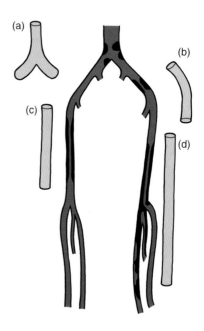

Figure 6.43 A schematic representation of approaches to bypass surgery, commonly used for macrovascular disease in diabetes. **(a)** Aorto-bifemoral. **(b)** Ilio-femoral. **(c)** Femoro-popliteal. **(d)** Femoro-distal.

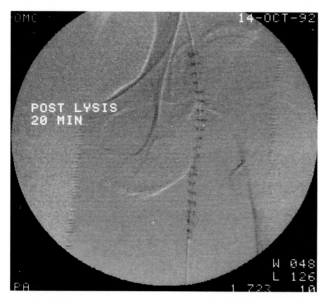

Figure 6.41 This digital subtraction image shows pulses of thrombolytic agent being sprayed from a catheter in the superficial femoral artery. Thrombolysis is especially valuable if it is felt that a stenosis is mainly the result of recent thrombus formation.

Figure 6.42(a) This X-ray shows good preservation of the popliteal and the trifurcation below the knee: ideal for bypass surgery to the superficial femoral artery. **(b)** In contrast, this shows appearances typical of diabetic macrovascular disease. It is usual to find very poor 'run-off' below the knee, with no major vessel available that might be used for the distal anastomosis.

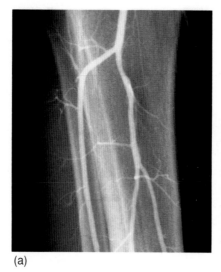

(a)

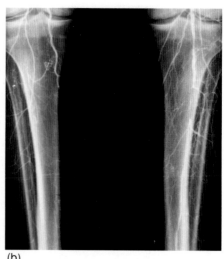

(b)

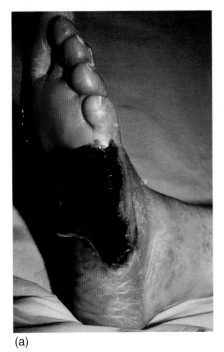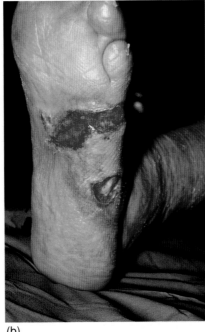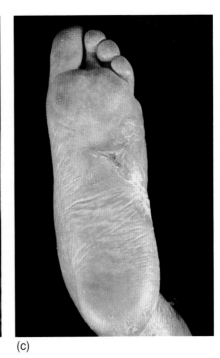

(a)   (b)   (c)

Figure 6.44(a) An extensive necrotic wound on the sole of the foot caused by a hot water bottle burn. **(b)** Long bypass surgery, using a graft from the superficial femoral to posterior tibial arteries resulted in revitalization of the tissue even though it was necessary to amputate the fifth toe. **(c)** The same foot, showing complete healing. This man was known to have a large-cell lung tumour at the time of his original presentation, but was treated nevertheless. He remains alive and well, with two feet.

Various materials can be used for the graft. Saphenous vein taken from the patient is used by preference but if no suitable vein is available an artificial graft is used. The usual choice is between Gortex and Dacron.

The outcome in those selected for bypass surgery is extremely good – both in terms of ulcer healing and limb salvage (Figure 6.44). This is so even though many grafts eventually become occluded by thrombus – presumably in such cases the graft served to maintain an effective circulation until such time as collaterals developed.

SKIN GRAFTING

Some chronic ulcers may be healed by skin grafting (Figure 6.45) and this is particularly useful in extensive ulcers of the shin – provided it is possible to eliminate superficial infection and slough (Figure 6.46). In general, however, most ulcers will heal without grafting provided that effective circulation can be established. In those that do not heal spontaneously, the graft often fails.

OTHER MEASURES

Healing is a complex process which requires an effective blood supply. When the blood supply is compromised, the therapeutic approaches are limited. Macrovascular flow might be improved, as described above, if the stenoses are few, short or bypassable. If they are distal, there is little that can be done. Similarly, there is nothing that can be done to reverse the effects of microvascular disease and attention must focus on:

1. regular cleansing to prevent secondary infection;
2. treatment of secondary infection when it occurs;
3. keeping pressure off the affected part by bed rest, padding and Scotchcast, or equivalent, techniques (see Chapter 7).

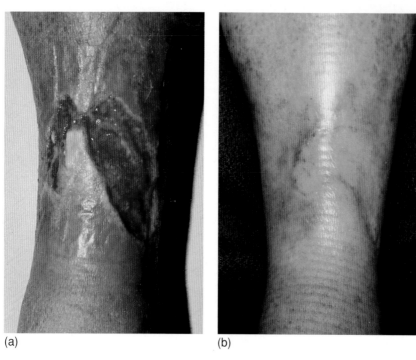

(a)

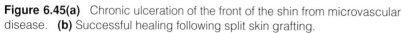

(b)

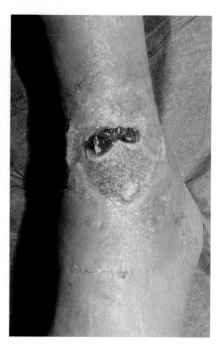

Figure 6.45(a) Chronic ulceration of the front of the shin from microvascular disease. **(b)** Successful healing following split skin grafting.

Figure 6.46 The soft black eschar and slough that forms on these superficial ulcers inhibits healing and must be removed – either piecemeal or under general anaesthesia.

7 Neuropathy

PATHOGENESIS

Diabetes leads to abnormal function of peripheral nerves for two main reasons: metabolic and ischaemic. Thus, high intracellular concentrations of glucose may be toxic to nerve cells – either directly, or indirectly through accumulation of sorbitol. Sorbitol is formed from glucose only when intracellular concentrations are excessive and saturate the normal glycolytic pathway (Figure 7.1).

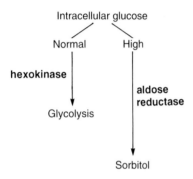

Figure 7.1 When concentrations of intracellular glucose are normal, then it is metabolized via the glycolytic pathway. If, however, they are high, glucose is converted by the enzyme aldose reductase into sorbitol.

However, it is likely that a more important reason for nerve damage in diabetes is ischaemia. Since nerves are dependent on the vasa nervorum for their nutrient supply, they will suffer ischaemic damage from microvascular disease (Figure 7.2). Neuropathy is always present in the grossly ischaemic leg.

While all nerves are affected, it is the longest – those to the feet – that are affected most. The clinical presentation depends on which nerve groups are involved.

TYPES OF PERIPHERAL NEUROPATHY

Sensory neuropathy

ANAESTHESIA

If the foot is anaesthetic because of neuropathy, the person may not notice trauma to the foot from, for instance, new shoes, a hot water bottle (Figure 7.3) or friction (Figure 7.4). In people with severe peripheral neuropathy, there may be sensory neuropathy also of the hands (Figure 7.5).

PAIN

Many people with diabetes have painful peripheral neuropathy as a result of neuropathy affecting small,

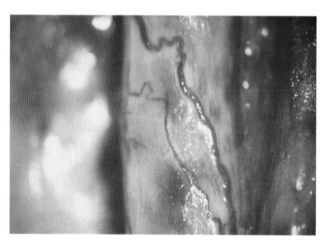

Figure 7.2 Disease of the vasa nervorum (the nutrient vessels of the nerves) is beautifully demonstrated in this illustration of a diabetic sural nerve (reproduced from Tesfaye, S., Harris, N., Jakubowski, J.J. *et al.* (1993) Impaired blood flow and arterio-venous shunting in human diabetic neuropathy: a novel technique of nerve photography and fluorescein angiography. Diabetologia, **36**: 1266, Figure 5, by kind permission of the publishers, Springer-Verlag).

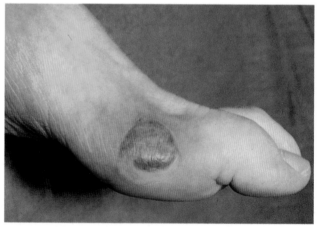

Figure 7.3 Burns on the foot from a hot water bottle. The patient was well aware of the risks, but the burns occurred even though the hot water bottle was covered with a woollen cosy.

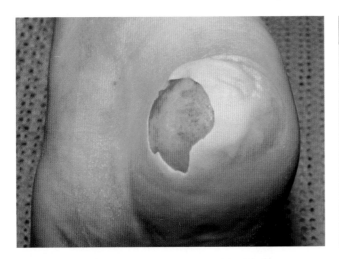

Figure 7.4 This heel ulcer was caused by friction on bedclothes and may have been the result of professional mismanagement. In the first 2 days after abdominal surgery the patient said she was instructed by a night-nurse to use her own heels to push herself upright in bed, and not to rely on being helped!

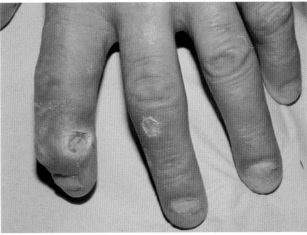

Figure 7.5 Peripheral neuropathy can affect the hands as well. This man did not notice that his cigarette was burning his fingers. He had had both his legs amputated for intractable infection complicating neuropathic ulcers of each leg in turn.

non-myelinated C fibres. This results in a persistent burning, aching or tingling feeling in the feet and lower leg – worst in bed at night (Figure 7.6).

In fact the risk of ulceration is less in people with painful peripheral neuropathy, possibly because their pain leads to greater awareness of the foot and hence to less risk of trauma. However, a difficulty can arise in attempting to determine whether pain in the foot of someone with an ulcer is the result of neuropathy, of infection or of critical ischaemia.

TEMPERATURE

There are two reasons why people might complain of having cold feet. The first is an abnormality of the nerve fibres carrying temperature sensation, such that the feet feel cold even though they are warm. The second is that the skin of the feet actually is abnormally cold – as a result either of macrovascular disease or of microvascular disease with abnormal shunting of blood away from the more superficial layers of skin (see Autonomic neuropathy, below).

Motor neuropathy

The integrity of the arch of the foot is preserved by muscles, ligaments and connective tissue. The muscles waste when affected by motor neuropathy – even though this may not be obvious because it is not easy to see the muscles of the normal foot. In addition, motor neuropathy causes loss of the normal balance between toe flexors and extensors and the

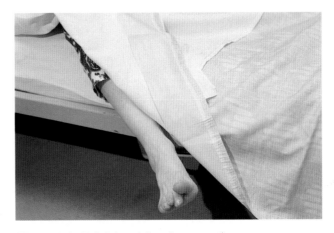

Figure 7.6 Painful peripheral neuropathy can cause considerable distress. The pain is often worst in bed, but it is not clear whether this is because the foot is elevated, or warmer, or whether it is simply because most pain seems worse at night. People derive relief from putting their feet out of the bedclothes and from letting them hang down.

person may develop either a flat foot, or one which is excessively clawed (Figure 7.7).

In either case there is redistribution of pressure under the sole and the load on certain points becomes excessive. This happens particularly over the head of the second metatarsal. The response of the skin to abnormal pressure is to thicken the layer of keratin as a protective mechanism, but this causes the development of callus (Figure 7.8).

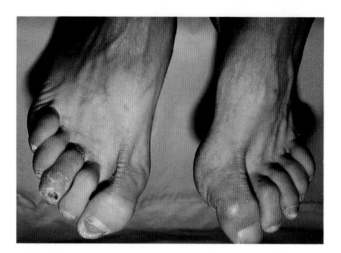

Figure 7.7 Exaggeration of the plantar arch and clawing of the toes are typical of peripheral motor neuropathy.

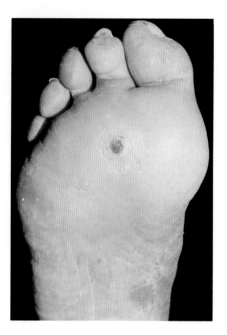

Figure 7.8 Increased pressure over the second metatarsal head causes build-up of callus which may then ulcerate.

Unfortunately the effect of the increased thickness of the callous skin on the foot (especially a foot in a shoe) is to increase the pressure loading still further (Figure 7.9). Eventually the loading leads to pressure necrosis and the area breaks down to produce the classical 'neuropathic' ulcer (Figure 7.10).

This process only happens if the blood supply to the foot is good enough to allow the build-up of callus. If the blood supply is poor, callus will not accumulate and the increase in pressure over the metatarsal head is then insufficient to cause ischaemic necrosis of the deeper tissues. In the ischaemic foot, ulceration occurs at points of more normal pressure loading – particularly at points where there are shearing forces, as over the medial

Figure 7.9 (right) Events leading to the development of a plantar neuropathic ulcer. **(a)** Exaggeration of the plantar arch and clawing of the toes results in excessive pressure being taken on the metatarsal heads and the toe tips, as well as the toe knuckles. This is unnoticed because of associated sensory neuropathy. **(b)** The accumulation of callus is primarily a protective process but in this case the result is to increase the pressure loading still further. **(c)** The increased pressure causes ischaemic necrosis of the tissues beneath the callus. **(d)** The callus breaks down to reveal a typical, clean, 'punched-out' neuropathic ulcer.

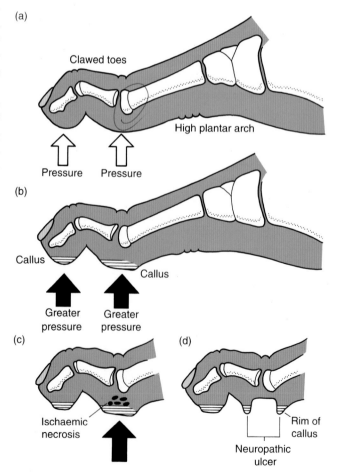

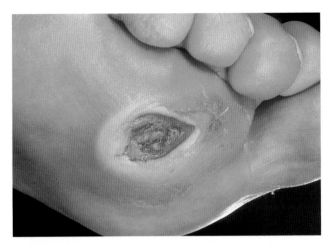

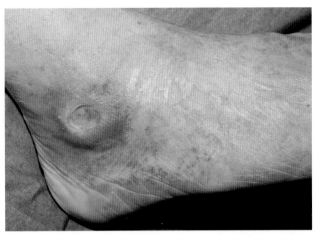

Figure 7.10 Typical plantar neuropathic ulcer which has developed because of pressure necrosis. The brown discoloration of surrounding skin is from povidone-iodine. Although these ulcers are normally benign, they are prone to secondary infection. This man was away on holiday when the ulcer became infected with *Clostridium perfringens*, and he died of gas gangrene. Infection with this organism is, fortunately, excessively rare – as it was even in Joslin's day (Chapter 1).

Figure 7.11 The 'neuroischaemic' ulcer develops at sites of more normal pressure loading in the foot in which both neuropathy and vasculopathy are moderately severe. It is clean and superficial but has less of the surrounding callus. Presumably the skin requires a good blood supply to build up sufficient callus to cause pressure necrosis as in Figure 7.10.

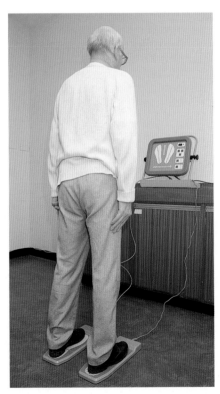

Figure 7.12 The combination of impaired proprioception and motor neuropathy leads to increased sway and imbalance which can be recorded, as here, with a balance platform.

aspect of the first metatarsophalangeal joint, the malleoli or between the toes. There is no surrounding callus. This is called a 'neuroischaemic' ulcer (Figure 7.11).

Proprioceptive loss

Although it has been little investigated, patients with neuropathy may also suffer loss of proprioception as a result of damage to the nerve fibres leading to the spinocerebellar pathways. This causes some degree of incoordination which will exacerbate the muscle imbalance caused by motor neuropathy (Figure 7.12).

Autonomic neuropathy

VASOMOTOR

The fine control of distribution of blood is dependent on the action of vasomotor nerves. These are responsible for opening and closing arterioles and venules such that blood is shunted to areas where it is most needed (Figure 7.13).

The result is that the foot affected by neuropathy may have abnormal distribution of blood within it: even though the macrovascular supply may be good, areas such as the skin may be relatively ischaemic. When the shunting from arteries to veins is gross, the foot pulses (dorsalis pedis, posterior tibial) are more

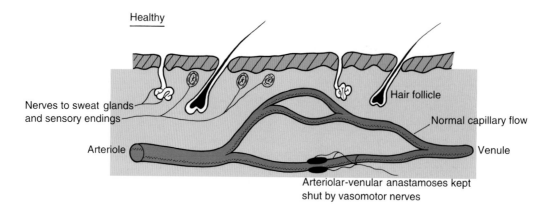

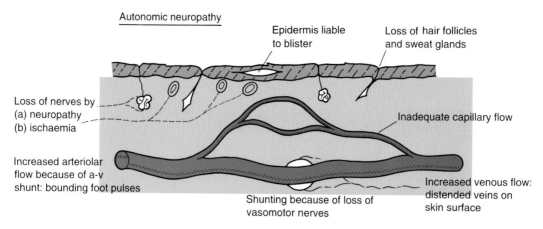

Figure 7.13 The neurotransmitters most involved in regulating distribution of blood within the microcirculation are not known, but the system is highly complex and dependent on autonomic innervation. Transmitters include noradrenaline, acetylcholine, nitric oxide, vasoactive intestinal polypeptide (VIP) and peptides derived from both the endothelium and other cells, such as endothelin, calcitonin gene-related peptide (CGRP), prostacyclin and thromboxane. When the autonomic nerve supply to the area is lost, there is no mechanism for distributing blood to the cells which need it most to maintain their integrity. The effects are summarized here.

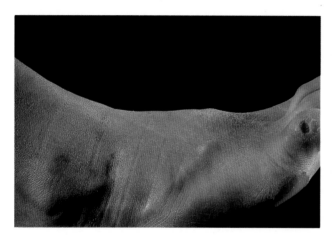

Figure 7.14 Distension of veins on the dorsum of the foot can be a sign of arteriovenous shunting from autonomic neuropathy. This patient also has a neuropathic ulcer on the fifth toe. Associated callus under the fifth metatarsal head has been well treated with chiropody.

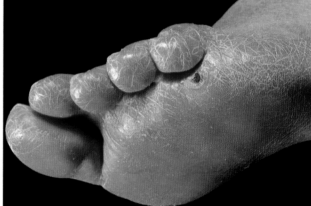

Figure 7.15 Dry and flaking skin results from a combination of autonomic denervation and ischaemia. The dry foot is particularly liable to ulceration and secondary infection.

easily felt than usual and the veins on the dorsum of the foot are distended (Figure 7.14). Failure of some chronic neuropathic ulcers to heal may be because autonomic neuropathy leads to reduced diversion of blood to the region of the ulcer, with reduced inflammation.

SWEATING

Loss of autonomic innervation leads to loss of sweating – both from loss of direct innervation, and from loss of skin blood flow (Figure 7.13). The skin becomes dry (Figure 7.15) and fissured; the normal skin flora is altered and there is increased risk of infection by pathogenic bacteria.

RECOGNITION OF NEUROPATHY

Inspection

While the foot with ischaemia has a thin, red, shiny skin, the neuropathic foot tends to look pale, podgy and hairless. The arch may be exaggerated and the toes clawed (Figure 7.16).

There is callus at points of increased pressure, particularly over the knuckles, the tips of the toes and the metatarsal heads on the sole (Figure 7.8). The abnormal distribution of weight may be apparent from examining the patient's shoes (Figure 7.17).

Muscle wasting may not be apparent in the foot affected by motor neuropathy but if any person has wasting of the small muscles of the hand it can be assumed that those in the foot are wasted as well (Figure 7.18).

Loss of hair growth is conventionally said to be a sign of severe vascular disease, but it actually reflects the presence of neuropathy more closely. Not only can people with bad vascular disease have persistent growth of hair on the toes (Figure 7.19), but hair is lost in the neuropathic foot with easily palpable pulses (Figure 7.20).

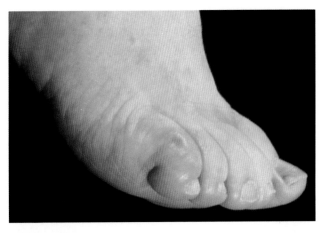

Figure 7.16 The foot affected by neuropathy is typically pale and puffy, with clawing of the toes and generalized thickening of the skin. This patient is at risk of developing a neuropathic ulcer over the fifth toe, as was the person in Figure 7.14.

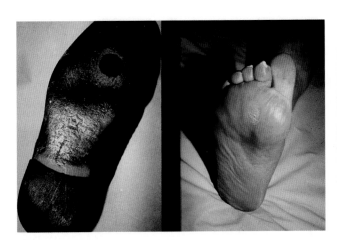

Figure 7.17 The increased pressure over the second metatarsal head is obvious from examining both the sole of the foot and the patient's shoe.

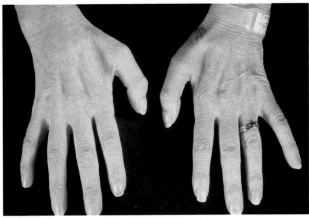

Figure 7.18 Wasting of the small muscles of the hands results in pronounced scalloping between the metacarpals. Any patient affected like this will also have muscle wasting in the feet – although it will not be so clinically obvious.

It is likely that this occurs because autonomic shunting of blood renders the skin and hair follicles relatively ischaemic – even though the overall supply of blood to the foot is good (Figure 7.13).

Examination

The most discriminant sign is loss of pin-prick sensation. This should be tested using a pin of the correct sharpness, such as a Neurotip (Figure 7.21), and not a venesection needle. Semi-quantitative assessment of pin-prick sensation can be obtained using monofilament hairs of differing grade: people with more severe neuropathy can feel only the coarser ones (Figure 7.22).

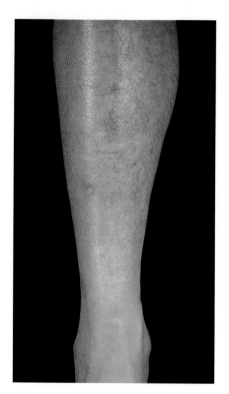

Figure 7.20   Hair loss on the lower leg is more usually a sign of neuropathy than of ischaemia, as shown in this illustration of the leg of a man in his 30s, the same person as in Figure 7.14. Hair has been lost from the shin and foot, but he has foot pulses which are easily felt. The foot is not ischaemic from macrovascular disease; it is the skin which is ischaemic from autonomic neuropathy.

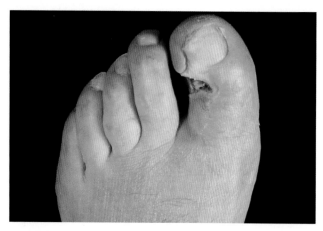

Figure 7.19   This man has severe peripheral vascular disease and has already had a below-knee amputation on the right. Note the persistence of hairs on the dorsum of the foot and toes.

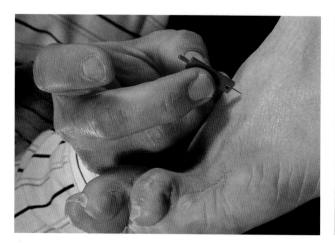

Figure 7.21   Examination for loss of pin-prick sensation is the most useful test in routine clinical practice.

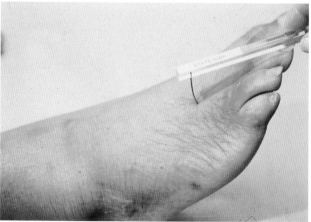

Figure 7.22   Semi-quantitative assessment of loss of pin-prick sensation can be obtained using monofilament variants of von Frey's hairs. The monofilament should be applied firmly enough to make it bend.

Testing for loss of soft touch is not of much value, because it tends to be preserved even in moderate to severe neuropathy. Similarly, there is little point in trying to elicit ankle reflexes, because they are almost uniformly absent in diabetics of this age group.

Vibration sense can be useful in detecting the younger person at risk of developing clinically significant neuropathy later. This can be done with a tuning fork (not higher than C128), but a semi-quantitative result is obtained using a Biothesiometer or equivalent device (Figure 7.23).

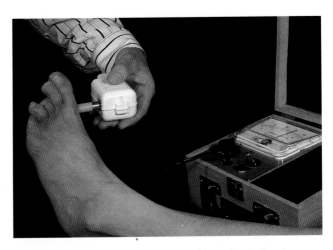

Figure 7.23 Clinical assessment of impaired vibration sense is not of much value partly because it is so common and partly because of the wide variance of clinical technique. The use of a Biothesiometer or equivalent device is better and may be a useful tool for detecting early the patient at particular risk of clinically significant neuropathy.

Testing for loss of temperature sensation is impractical, while the only tests available for autonomic neuropathy are tests of vasomotor control of cardiac and large vessel function and not really relevant.

PEDOBAROGRAPHY

Some specialist units have employed computerized methods to demonstrate points of high pressure under the sole (Figure 7.24).

Non-computerized methods, such as the Harris mat, are also available. However, all these techniques are relatively expensive and not necessary in routine clinical practice.

MANAGEMENT OF THE NEUROPATHIC FOOT AT RISK OF ULCERATION

Definition of the 'at risk' foot

It is known that someone with clinical evidence of neuropathy (loss of pin-prick sensation; abnormal Biothesiometer recording) has a much increased risk of ulceration in the succeeding 5 years. They have to be told that their foot is at risk, and told how to minimize the chance of unnoticed trauma from, for example, new shoes. They need to examine their feet daily and, if the skin is dry, to use hand cream or E45 to try to make it more supple. Most important of all, they need to seek help at the first sign of trouble.

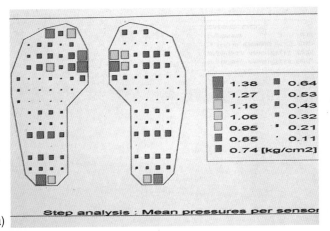

(a)

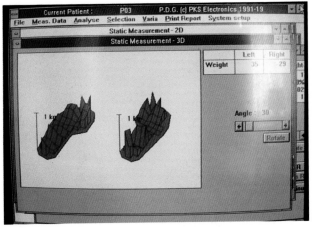

(b)

Figure 7.24(a) A computerized pedobarograph which records pressures under the sole both while the patient is standing still and during walking. This particular method employs sensors embedded within insoles designed to fit inside the patient's shoe. **(b)** The two pedobarograph print-outs show particularly increased force being exerted on the heel and when walking (lower figure) over the first metatarsal head and tips of the first and second toes on the left.

The 'at risk' foot should be clearly defined in clinical records (Figure 7.25), and the professional should make a point of examining 'at risk' feet at least each year.

Reducing abnormal pressure

CHIROPODY

Neuropathic ulceration is triggered by the build-up of callus at points of abnormally high pressure. This can usually be prevented if the callus is removed regularly by a chiropodist. This needs to be done each 3–4 weeks in someone with good blood supply to their feet, but the accumulation of callus is less marked with increasing degrees of ischaemia. The effect of chiropody in reducing pressure is shown in Figure 7.26. For further details, see Chapter 9.

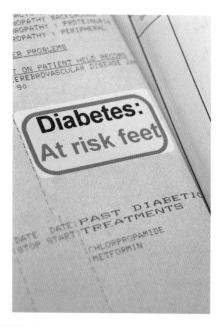

Figure 7.25 Medical and nursing records should be clearly flagged to draw attention to a problem which might not otherwise be emphasized.

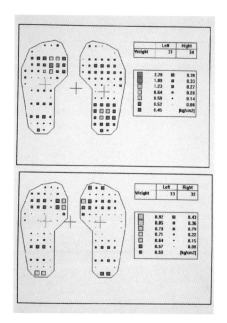

Figure 7.26 These two pedobarography traces demonstrate the effect of chiropody in reducing the high pressure being exerted through the metatarsal heads. If the pressure can be kept down in this way, the skin will not ulcerate.

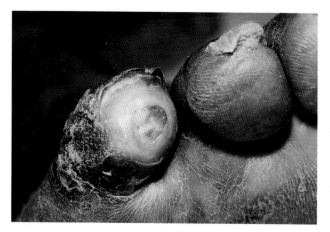

Figure 7.27 Neuropathic ulceration on the tip of a clawed toe.

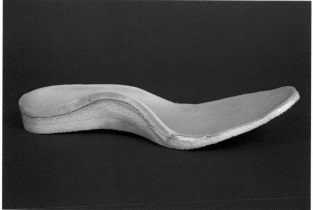

Figure 7.28 Fitted footwear should incorporate generous instep support where necessary, and the shoe itself should be deep and roomy enough to accommodate the foot without being so floppy that it predisposes to shearing stress.

FOOTWEAR

Footwear can be chosen to reduce points of high pressure – both under the sole and elsewhere. In most cases the problem is caused by the arching of the foot, with more plantar pressure being taken under the metatarsal heads (Figure 7.8). Callus may also accumulate on the tips of the toes, leading to ulceration if untreated (Figure 7.27). Fitted shoes should have generous instep support to distribute the weight more evenly over the sole (Figure 7.28).

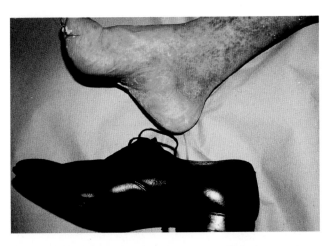

Figure 7.29 Many people have an unrealistic impression of the extent of the deformity of their feet, leading to the use of inappropriate footwear. This is made worse by the pressure of fashion and the difficulty in finding shoes of the right shape on sale.

The other problem of clawing is that there is an increased requirement for a deep shoe – to prevent the knuckles of the toes rubbing on the top of the shoe. The situation is made worse if people have an uncompromising allegiance to the dictates of fashion (Figure 7.29).

The principle of fitted footwear is to provide a shoe which is deep enough and broad enough, but not floppy. The material should be soft, and there should be good instep support. Suitable shoes may be chosen by the patient, or may need to be provided by an orthotist. If the latter, the patient may have a stock shoe with a tailored insole (cost about £50), or have one made to measure (cost up to £400) (Figures 7.30 and 7.31).

It is not enough, however, simply to provide shoes. They need to be worn as well. They need to be checked regularly and must be repaired and replaced when necessary: there is little to be gained by simply going through the motions of ulcer prevention by providing a single pair of shoes on a single occasion (Figure 7.32). This subject is also covered in Chapter 12.

PROTECTION IN HOSPITALS

All professionals concerned with management need to be aware of the risks to the neuropathic foot – especially those caring for the person when they are immobilized through illness. The heels, in particular, need regular checking and protection (Figure 7.33). This subject is discussed in more detail in Chapter 12.

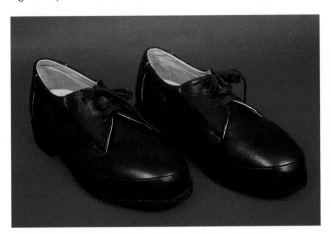

Figure 7.30 A stock shoe available from orthotic suppliers which is deep enough to accomodate insoles fitted to the shape of the patient's foot.

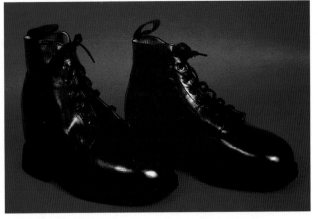

Figure 7.31 Bespoke footwear may be needed for feet which are particularly deformed, especially following Charcot arthropathy, but such shoes are expensive.

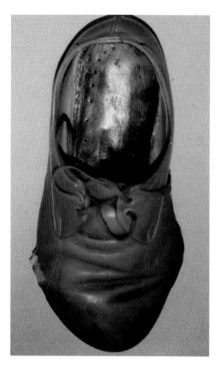

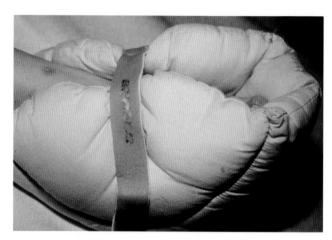

Figure 7.32 Provision of fitted footwear is an open-ended commitment. It is not enough to provide a single pair of shoes on a single occasion – especially, as here, to someone who may not realise the need to request more when the old ones have ceased to serve their purpose. The insole had apparently been chewed by the patient's dog, and so she had gone without.

Figure 7.33 Heels should be protected – especially in those with severe peripheral vascular disease. There is no ideal method available and although the padded boot illustrated may protect the heel, it is difficult to pad about in, difficult to keep in place and may be hot and uncomfortable.

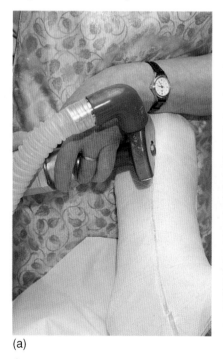

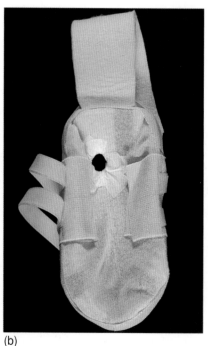

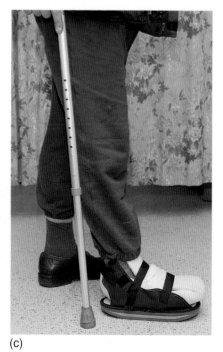

(a)   (b)   (c)

Figure 7.34(a) The Scotchcast boot is moulded to the whole foot before the top is removed. A hole is cut over the position of the ulcer – in order to alleviate the pressure at that point. **(b)** The half-boot is then padded and provided with Velcro straps to hold it in place. This shows the window which has been left over the heel to take pressure off an ulcer. **(c)** An overshoe can be supplied to enable the patient to get about and do essential chores.

MANAGEMENT OF NEUROPATHIC ULCERATION

The principles of management of any ulcer are those which have been set out in Chapters 3–6. The first priority is to treat any infection that is present and the second is to define any vasculopathy. If there is clinical evidence of macrovascular disease, angiography should be considered. Thereafter the main aim of management is to alleviate the pressure which caused the problem as well as to keep the ulcer clean in order to promote healing.

Alleviation of pressure

Bed rest is important if the ulcer is infected, but impractical if it is not. The median healing time is 12 weeks for an uncomplicated neuropathic ulcer and it is neither feasible nor desirable for a person to rest in bed for that length of time. Therefore, they should be asked to keep their weight off the foot as much as possible and, if they are ambulant, they should have a walking plaster.

WALKING PLASTER: THE REMOVABLE SCOTCHCAST BOOT

The principle of the removable boot is that it is padded to deflect pressure from the ulcerated part. Although it is cumbersome (and there is a risk that some elderly people may be made unsteady by one), it is light and easily removed for cleaning and dressing of the ulcer and for going to bed (Figure 7.34). An overshoe is provided for going outside.

There are a number of variants, and these devices can be used to take pressure off ischaemic ulcers as well. Those with windows in the heel are especially useful for nursing heel ulcers in the patient who is largely immobilized through ill health.

WALKING PLASTER: TOTAL CONTACT CAST

An alternative approach is to encase the foot in a total contact cast which is not removable by the patient (Figure 7.35).

This is only appropriate if there is no clinical evidence of infection. The cast is usually removed each week. Those with slough and dirty wounds need regular cleansing and debridement (Chapter 10). However, others use below-knee casts of this type, in which a window is cut to allow wound cleaning. Alternatively, a full-length below-knee cast can be split down the side: it provides firmer support while walking, but is still removable at night (Figure 7.36).

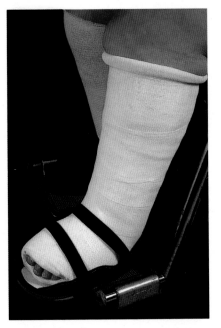

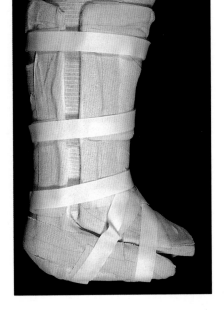

Figure 7.35 (left) Intractable neuropathic ulceration is better managed with a total contact cast – suitably padded to protect the ulcer from pressure. The cast is removed weekly to check for infection and to change dressings.

Figure 7.36 (right) A total contact cast can be split down its length so that it can be taken off at night.

NEUROPATHIC OSTEOARTHROPATHY – CHARCOT JOINT

Jean-Martin Charcot was the first Professor of Diseases of the Nervous System at the Salpêtrière in Paris and his recognition of the association between disease of the nervous system and gross disorganization of the joints of the spine and lower limb led to the latter being termed 'Charcot's joint' in 1882 (Figure 7.37).

Charcot's belief was that disease of the nervous system led to the collapse of the bones and joints because of interruption of their normal nutritive supply. On the other hand the 'German school' of the time maintained that the bones collapsed simply because they were anaesthetic through impairment of deep pain sensation and hence subjected by the patient to chronic unnoticed trauma. Most modern physicians subscribe to the German theory, but it is increasingly recognized that Charcot was probably

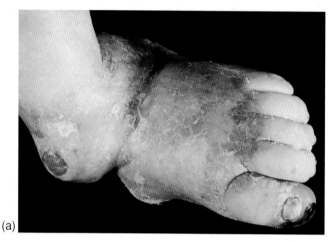

(a)

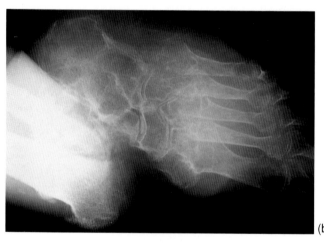

(b)

Figure 7.37(a) Destruction of the ankle joint caused by diabetic (Charcot) neuropathic osteoarthropathy. Deformity of this severity will be associated with intractable ulceration

and secondary infection, and amputation may be necessary even though the circulation to the limb is good and there is little risk of gangrene. **(b)** X-ray appearance of **(a)**.

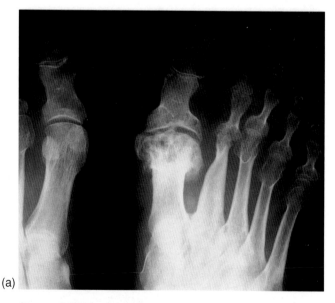

(a)

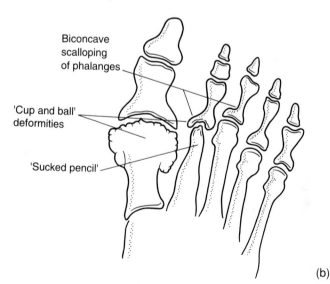

(b)

Figure 7.38(a) Typical radiological features of osteoarthropathy in the digits: biconcave scalloping of the phalanges and erosion of the heads of the metatarsals

('sucked pencil') and 'cup and ball' deformities of the metatarsophalangeal joints. **(b)** Diagrammatic illustration of **(a)**.

right – at least in diabetes: it is not painlessness which leads to the destruction of the bones and joints, but an underlying change in the strength and integrity of bone structure resulting from neuropathy. In this respect the processes leading to the development of Charcot deformity in diabetes may be crucially different from those in leprosy, syringomyelia and tabes dorsalis.

Pathogenesis

Diabetics with peripheral neuropathy but without gross macrovascular disease have been shown to have increased blood flow to the feet, caused by autonomic neuropathy with increased arteriovenous shunting. The foot pulses are easily palpable and the venous oxygen content is high. It is thought that it is this increase in blood flow which leads to the bone changes: there is increased bone turnover (with increased uptake in three-phase technetium scans) with net loss of bone matrix.

OSTEOARTHROPATHY IN THE METATARSALS AND PHALANGES

When these changes occur in the smaller bones of the foot, the metatarsals and phalanges, they are seen on X-ray to be thinned and deformed. Patchy lucency occurs and the head of the metatarsal typically becomes tapered, like a 'sucked pencil'. There is erosion of the articular cartilage. The base of the phalanx may become widened and the metatarsophalangeal joint look like a 'cup and ball' (Figure 7.38). The metatarsophalangeal and interphalangeal joints may dislocate (Figures 7.39 and 7.40).

After the acute phase of bone destruction the bones go through a sclerotic phase and new bone formation is seen, with exostoses (Figure 7.41). Any of these deformities may be complicated by secondary neuropathic ulceration of the toes.

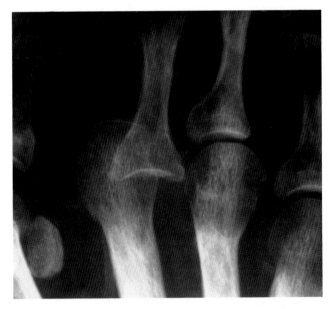

Figure 7.39 Dislocation of the second metatarsophalangeal joint in diabetic arthropathy.

Figure 7.40(a) X-ray of the foot showing normal tarso-metatarsal (Lisfranc) joints. **(b)** The same foot, showing Lisfranc disarticulation, with lateral displacement of the bases of the metatarsals.

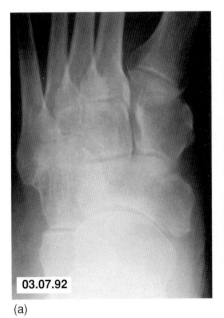

03.07.92

(a)

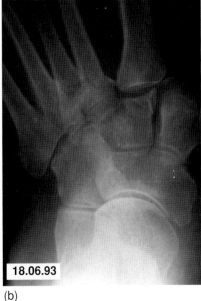

18.06.93

(b)

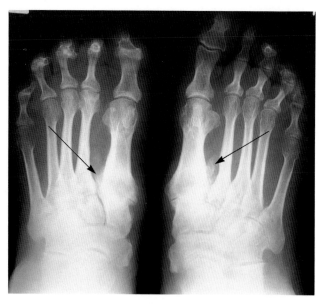

Figure 7.41 Exostoses, seen arrowed here at the base of each first metatarsal, appear during the phase of sclerosis and reossification.

OSTEOARTHROPATHY IN THE TARSAL BONES

When this process affects the larger bones of the foot and ankle, the destruction and deformity is greater, because the forces acting on the weakened bones are considerable. Thus, it is not unusual to record pressures of 5–10 kg/cm² under the metatarsal heads during walking; the weight of the whole body acts through the tibiotalar and subtalar joints. The start of the deformity may occur in response to unnoticed or to trivial trauma, such as tripping over an object on the floor. However, the minor deformity caused by the injury increases local disruptive forces, leading to further disorganization, and a vicious cycle is triggered. The bones collapse and the whole shape of the foot alters – usually with loss of the arch and medial bulging (Figure 7.42).

When the deformity is complicated by neuropathic ulceration, there may be secondary infection and the osteomyelitis leads to further destruction. Osteomyelitis in a Charcot foot can be impossible to eradicate.

Table 7.1 Processes involved in the development of diabetic neuropathic osteoarthropathy

1. Autonomic neuropathy leads to arteriovenous shunting with overall increased blood flow through the foot.

2. The increased blood flow causes, or is associated with, increased bone turnover with net loss of bone.

3. The smaller bones of the foot show lucency and tapering of the metatarsals.

4. Various factors lead to traumatic injury to the weakened bones – forces during normal walking; increased forces resulting from motor neuropathy and limited joint mobility; or an accident.

5. Some injuries are chronic and not grossly destructive, such as the 'cup and ball' deformity of the metatarsophalangeal joint (Figure 7.38), dislocation of the metatarsophalangeal joint or lateral dislocation of the tarsometatarsal joints (Lisfranc disarticulation) (Figure 7.40).

6. Other injuries cause deformity which leads to a critical increase in local forces, leading in turn to progressive deformity of the structure of the bones. This is seen most frequently when the process affects the tarsal bones – the cuneiforms, cuboid, navicular, calcaneum and talus.

7. The disorganized bone starts to repair with increasing sclerosis on X-ray, with exostoses resulting from new bone laid down by torn and displaced periosteum (Figure 7.41).

8. In the chronic phase, there is no further destruction of bone and the foot loses its hyperaemic warmth. The original deformity persists, however, and there is a great risk of secondary neuropathic ulceration of skin over abnormal bony prominences. Any ulceration can be complicated by osteomyelitis.

The process of diabetic neuropathic osteoarthropathy

The process is summarized in Table 7.1.

The foot, which is predisposed to the changes by autonomic neuropathy with hyperaemia and thinning of bones, undergoes progressive destruction and deformity over a period of months. This is made worse if the skin ulcerates and the bone becomes infected. If this does not happen, the foot eventually stabilizes and the bones reossify (Figure 7.41).

It is curious that the process of diabetic neuro-osteoarthropathy usually proves self-limiting: one would expect the dissolution of bone to be progressive if it was caused by hyperaemia from irreversible autonomic neuropathy. It is possible that this happens because the degree of arteriovenous shunting lessens in some way as the neuropathy worsens, or it is possible that the increased blood supply is eventually reduced by the onset of macrovascular disease. It is also possible, and perhaps most likely, that the autonomic hyperaemia is itself an uncoordinated response to another stimulus. If the hyperaemia was itself triggered by, for example, an ulcer or infection in the foot, then this would explain its transience.

Recognition

ASYMPTOMATIC

Chronic changes in the metatarsals and phalanges may be noted on X-ray, as well as dislocation of minor joints which may not be clinically obvious.

ACUTE

During the acute phase the patient will usually complain of a swollen, red, painful foot – which may follow noticed trauma or may seem to be spontaneous. Clinically, it may be indistinguishable from sprain, small fracture, cellulitis or gout – although neither pain nor tenderness are severe (Figure 5.20(a)). There may be a joint effusion and ligaments may be noted to be lax. Charcot arthropathy is bilateral in 10–20% of cases and the diagnosis should be strongly suspected if a patient who already has a stable deformity in one foot develops tender redness of the other.

DESTRUCTIVE

Once the structure of the tarsal bones becomes disorganized, the diagnosis is obvious. The only difficulty lies in distinguishing Charcot arthropathy from osteomyelitis, and if the skin is broken and there is a real possibility of bone infection, it can be impossible to distinguish between them (Figures 5.20 and 7.43(a)). If the skin is broken, the patient may well have both (Figure 7.43(b)).

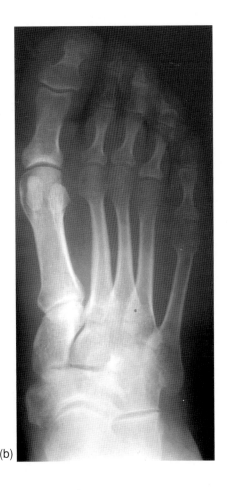

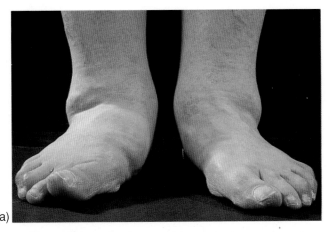

(a)

Figure 7.42(a) Feet distorted by osteoarthropathy, with medial bulging of the tarsus and loss of the plantar arch. **(b)** X-ray of the right foot of the patient shown in Figure 7.41 and in **(a)**. It was taken 7 years earlier and is normal.

(b)

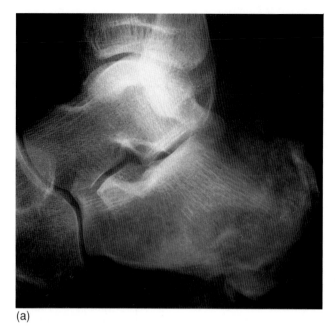

(a)

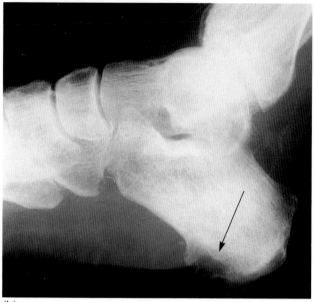

(b)

Figure 7.43(a) Plain X-ray of the heel of the man whose heel is illustrated in Figure 5.20(a). The calcaneum is starting to disintegrate as a result of diabetic neuropathic osteoarthropathy. Although the appearance is compatible with bone infection, there was no other clinical, biochem- ical or radiological (Figure 5.20(b)) evidence of osteomyelitis. **(b)** In another case, a deep, penetrating ulcer in the soft tissues beneath the calcaneum led to secondary osteomyelitis. This proved impossible to eradicate, and the leg was lost.

Investigations

In the acute phase the first object of investigation is to exclude fracture, cellulitis and gout. Positive diagnosis of neuropathic osteoarthropathy can be more difficult: the white cell count is normal, as is the C-reactive protein. The sedimentation rate (ESR) may be normal or slightly raised. An elevated alkaline phosphatase would suggest osteomyelitis rather than uninfected osteoarthropathy. Confirmation of the diagnosis is radiological.

PLAIN X-RAY

The bones are typically lucent, but this may not be particularly apparent in the acute phase. In the phase of destruction there is progressive disruption and distortion, with new bone formation in the later stages.

COMPUTED TOMOGRAPHY (CT) AND MAGNETIC RESONANCE IMAGING (MRI)

CT scanning will reveal changes in both soft tissues and bone and may help in distinguishing uninfected osteoarthropathy from osteomyelitis. MRI may also be used to establish the primary diagnosis, and typical T_1- and T_2-weighted images have been described.

BONE BIOPSY

There is no place in routine practice for bone biopsy to establish or exclude the presence of infection. The risk of introducing bacteria into non-infected bone outweighs the advantages. If the presence of infection is seriously considered, it should simply be treated.

ISOTOPE SCANS

Increased uptake of tracer can be demonstrated in affected bone, whether technetium or gallium is used (Figure 7.44).

Such scans are of little value, however, in differentiating osteoarthropathy from osteomyelitis because bone uptake occurs in both. Nevertheless, a positive diagnosis of bone infection can be made by scanning with leucocytes labelled with indium or technetium tracer, which carries a diagnostic specificity of approximately 90% (Figure 5.20(b)).

Management of acute neuropathic osteoarthropathy

IMMOBILIZATION AND WEIGHT-SPARING

Once the acute destructive phase is recognized, the objective is to reduce eventual deformity by removing as much pressure as possible from the foot. This needs to be continued until the clinical signs have resolved – there is no pain, the skin is less warm and the swelling is much reduced – which may not be for 2–3 months.

The foot should be immobilized in a below-knee plaster and weight bearing should be strictly limited by the use of rest, crutches and wheelchair. If this is achieved, the long-term benefit may be considerable because recurrent ulceration is much less likely if the final foot deformity is slight.

BIPHOSPHONATES

Biphosphonates are chelating agents which bind to bone and stabilize the crystal lattice, and are widely used in the management of Paget's disease. The administration of biphosphonates, such as pamidronate, by infusion during the acute phase of osteoarthropathy has been reported to cause arrest of the destructive process. If a positive diagnosis of acute osteoarthropathy is made, biphosphonates should probably be given but more evidence is required from controlled trials.

Management of chronic deformity

The risk is of recurrent neuropathic ulceration and if this is complicated by deep infection the ulcer may never heal. Hence the chance of ulceration must be reduced by:

1. regular chiropody to remove callus;
2. provision of footwear – which needs to be bespoke (Figure 7.45);
3. surgical correction of residual deformity in some cases, but only when the disease has entered the quiescent phase;
4. amputation of the limb, which may prove necessary if the process is complicated by osteomyelitis; this is often the correct course in the younger patient immobilized by recurrent infection and ulceration (Figure 7.46).

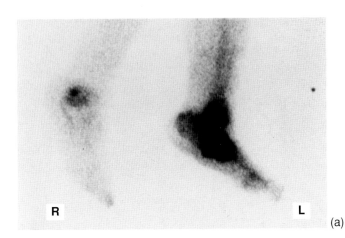

(a)

Figure 7.44(a) A late-phase bone scan using biphosphonate labelled with technetium as tracer. There is increased uptake in both feet, but especially on the left. The appearance on the left suggests marked destruction of the tarsal bones. A bone scan like this does not differentiate between neuropathic osteoarthropathy and osteomyelitis. **(b)** Further scans, showing uptake also in the right knee. This was thought to be the result of a stress fracture from abnormal weightbearing caused by the need to rest the left foot. There is also uptake in the bladder, which is expected, from excretion of isotope.

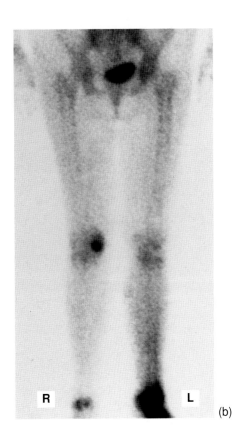

(b)

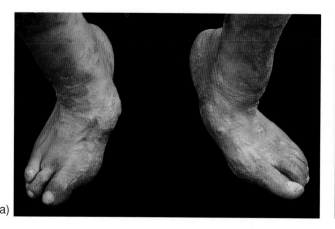

(a)

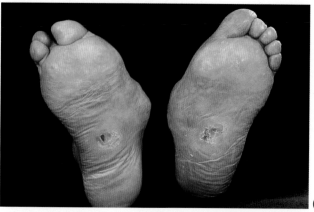

(b)

Prevention

At the moment it is not possible to prevent the onset of neuropathic osteoarthropathy, but it may at some stage be possible to identify a group at particular risk – perhaps the younger patient with peripheral neuropathy and, for example, distended foot veins. If so, it may become normal practice to treat with biphosphonates if increased bone turnover is demonstrated by technetium scan or by detecting an increase in osteocalcin or urinary hydroxyproline.

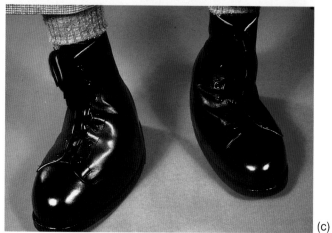

(c)

Figure 7.45(a) Gross bilateral deformity resulting from Charcot arthropathy. **(b)** The deformity leads to accumulation of callus and to secondary neuropathic ulceration at points of high pressure. This may occur over the medial bulge, or over the flattened instep, as shown here. **(c)** Shoes made to measure for the patient whose feet are illustrated in **(a)** and **(b)**.

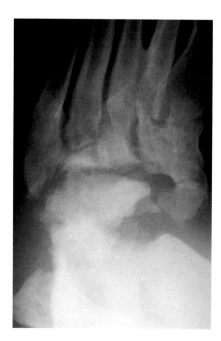

Figure 7.46 The gross destruction of the ankle joint and lower leg which resulted from a combination of osteoarthropathy and osteomyelitis (see also Figure 3.9). Cure is often impossible, and it is best to proceed to early below-knee amputation.

8 Skin and nail conditions

Diabetes can cause changes in the skin and nails of the feet because of neuropathy, vasculopathy and underlying alterations in the structure of the connective tissue. The pathogenesis is not always clearly defined.

SKIN CONDITIONS ASSOCIATED WITH DIABETES

Dry skin

Loss of autonomic innervation of sweat glands may render the surface of the foot dry (Figure 8.1). Coupled with alterations in epidermal elasticity and thinning of the skin (Figure 8.2), splits occur which form sites for entry of pathogenic bacteria (Figure 8.3).

Skin cracks due to dryness are commonest around the heel and should be dealt with by twice daily application of an emollient cream such as E45 after washing. This may or may not prevent deterioration, but it will certainly ensure that the feet are inspected regularly.

Necrobiosis lipoidica diabeticorum

Necrobiosis occurs in about 1% of diabetics and may predate the onset of the disease (Figure 8.4).

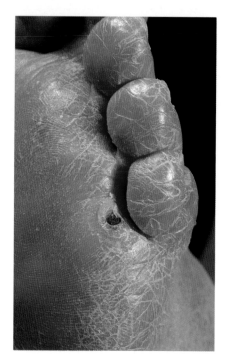

Figure 8.1 Autonomic neuropathy leads to loss of normal sweating, which leaves the skin dry and flaking. When this is associated with peripheral vascular disease, as here, the skin is also thin, atrophic and susceptible to trauma. In addition there is an infarct (which was typically painful) under the fifth toe, caused by occlusion of a small end-artery.

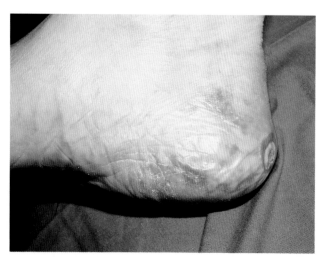

Figure 8.2 The heel of the dry, ischaemic foot is similarly atrophic. A sloughy ulcer has been rubbed on the back of it.

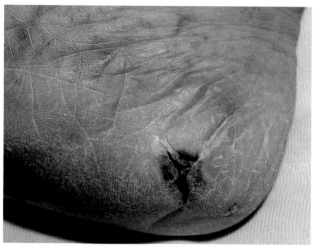

Figure 8.3 Deep fissuring of the skin acts a portal for pathogenic bacteria. When fissuring is associated with small areas of infarction within the dermis, it can be very painful.

Women are affected four times more often than men. In the early phases it occurs on the shins as irregular, raised, erythematous plaques which include deposits of extracellular fat. These atrophy from the centre outwards leaving thin brownish areas which tend to coalesce. These persist indefinitely and are unsightly but painless, unless they ulcerate and become infected (see Figure 5.12). There is no treatment other than protection from trauma and management of any ulceration that occurs.

Eruptive xanthomata

People with diabetes are at risk of hyperlipidaemia, and rarely this may be gross. Such severe combined hypercholesterolaemia and hypertriglyceridaemia is a feature of certain patients with non-insulin dependent diabetes caused by marked insulin resistance, and they may present with eruptive xanthomata (Figure 8.5).

Macrophages filled with lipid are deposited on the surface of the skin to form fleshy, raised, pink and yellow nodules with irregular margins. These respond to a combination of diet and lipid-lowering agents, and insulin may be indicated – even though they are not strictly insulin-dependent.

Diabetic dermopathy

Diabetic dermopathy (Figure 8.6) is probably the commonest cutaneous condition associated with diabetes.

Its cause is unknown. It occurs on the shins and dorsal surface of the foot, and is twice as common in men as in women. It appears as discrete, scattered, brown, slightly depressed areas. There is no treatment and it persists indefinitely.

Granuloma annulare

Granuloma annulare is thought to be more common in diabetes, even though it is seen only rarely (Figure 8.7).

It is caused by granulomatous infiltration within the dermis and is histologically indistinguishable

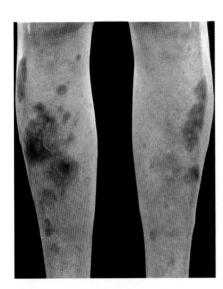

Figure 8.4 Necrobiosis lipoidica diabeticorum leaves large, semi-coalescent areas of thinned, brownish skin – usually on the front of the shins.

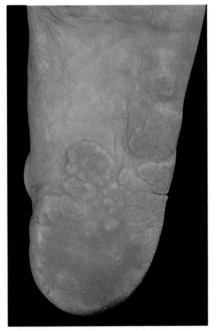

Figure 8.5 Eruptive xanthomata occur in gross combined hyperlipidaemia (elevation of both cholesterol and triglycerides), which is a rare manifestation of non-insulin-dependent diabetes with marked insulin resistance. The fatty deposits may be itchy, and may be found anywhere on the body, including the feet.

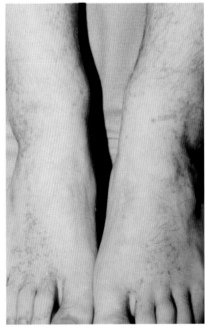

Figure 8.6 Diabetic dermopathy is the name given to the multiple brown atrophic spots which look like large freckles and are commonly seen on the shins of people with diabetes. The cause is unknown.

from necrobiosis lipoidica diabeticorum. The palpable, pinkish nodules form annular or arc-like lesions with flattened centres. Apart from being disfiguring, the condition is asymptomatic and benign and the lumps tend to fade with the passage of time.

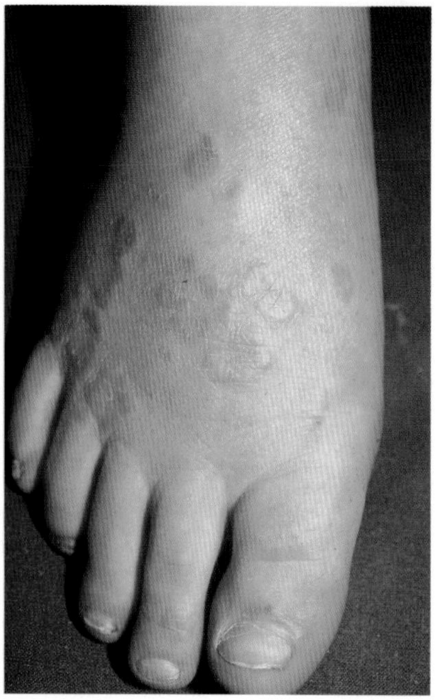

Lichen planus

The lesions of lichen planus are itchy, bluish, flat-topped papules which are seen most commonly on the forearms and shins. It is possibly more common in diabetes, but the aetiology is unknown. It responds to treatment with topical steroids.

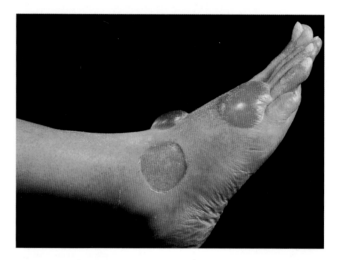

Figure 8.7 Granuloma annulare is a rare disorder which is thought to be more common in diabetes. The lesions are typically raised, pale and painless. The condition is indistinguishable histologically from necrobiosis lipoidica diabeticorum.

Figure 8.8 Diabetic blisters (bullosis diabeticorum) occur because the skin is ischaemic with loss of the normal fibrous bands (anchoring fibrils) which bind epidermis and dermis together. The blisters are caused by minor shearing forces such as movement of the foot against bedclothes. It is usually seen in patients with severe cardiac and peripheral vascular disease, as here, but a slightly different form is seen in those with autonomic neuropathy (see Figure 8.9).

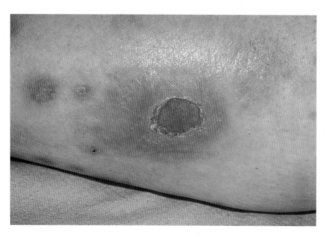

Figure 8.9 Patients with autonomic neuropathy may have abnormal shunting of blood to the skin as a result of arterio-venous anastomoses. The result is that some areas are relatively ischaemic and may blister or undergo infarction. The lesion usually starts as a raised, itchy lump which may or may not become a frank blister or break down. It heals leaving a scar. These lesions occur either singly or in crops and are most often seen in those with associated diabetic renal damage.

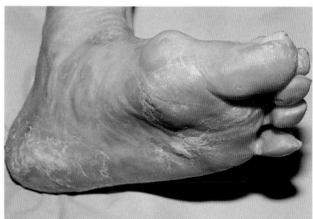

Figure 8.10 There is increased build-up of callus as a result of psoriasis.

Bullosis diabeticorum

Spontaneous blistering of the skin, or blistering in response to minor shearing forces, is a recognized feature of diabetes. It indicates premature ageing of skin, with loss of the normal anchoring fibrils in the epidermis, and is caused by relative skin ischaemia. It is seen most often in those with cardiac and peripheral vascular disease and poor peripheral perfusion (Figure 8.8). It is best managed by simple exposure to the air. If blisters burst, they need dressing with non-adherent dressings such as paratulle.

Blistering may also be seen in those with autonomic neuropathy and altered vasomotor control of the microcirculation of the skin. Such people may also suffer recurrent crops of small, itchy lumps which may appear anywhere on the body, occasionally break down and scab, but eventually heal with a small scar (Figure 8.9). This is likely to be the result of microvascular disease. Affected patients are often thought, wrongly, to have dermatitis artefacta (see Figure 8.15).

Hyperkeratosis from psoriasis

Psoriasis is no more common in people with diabetes than it is in those without, but its occurrence may exacerbate any tendency to build-up of neuropathic callus: it is a disease characterized by hyperkeratosis that is most marked in areas of increased pressure (Figure 8.10).

It should be considered in any patient with unusual build-up of skin around a lesion, and there may be tell-tale signs of the disease elsewhere, with characteristic red patches with raised margins and silvery scales on the surface. Nails may be pitted or thickened or discoloured. Chiropody will be required, but steroid creams may also be considered if the build-up of callus interferes with management.

TRAUMA

Simple skin abrasions occur more frequently in diabetic patients. As previously noted, autonomic

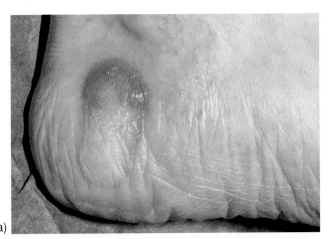 (a)
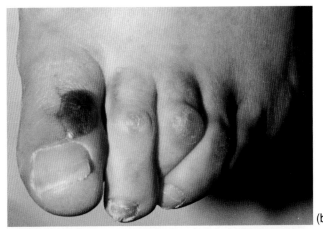 (b)
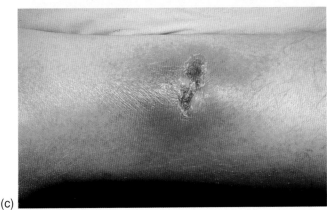 (c)
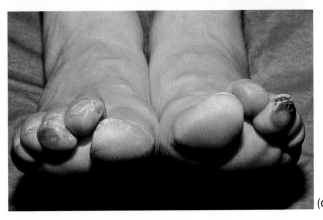 (d)

Figure 8.11(a) This blister was caused by a burn from a hot water bottle. It occurred despite the bottle being in a woollen cover. **(b)** A blood blister on the hallux, probably caused by wearing shoes that were too tight. The patient had also developed corns over the deformity of her toes for the same reason. **(c)** A blister caused by rubbing from a work boot, which was unnoticed because of peripheral neuropathy. **(d)** Blisters on the ends of the toes caused by sitting in front of a fan-heater.

neuropathy leads to anhidrosis, which makes the skin of the foot less resistant to damage. Sensory neuropathy means that if an accident occurs the person may not realize anything has happened, or they may only notice that their shoes are rubbing after a break in the skin has been made. A variety of blisters due to trauma are shown in Figure 8.11.

Simple abrasions, if unattended, may deteriorate in those with poor peripheral circulation, and it is those with poor circulation who are most likely to damage the skin from minor injury. If abrasions become infected, there may be disastrous results. It is important to stress the need for urgent professional advice to those with an 'at risk' foot – even though an injury may appear trivial.

Dermatitis artefacta

Dermatitis artefacta is the name given to repeated self-inflicted trauma caused by picking and scratching (Figure 8.12).

It occurs most often in the simple-minded, but may be a presentation of an attention-seeking illness.

The lesions are usually multiple and widespread, with no apparent cause, and will heal rapidly when protected. It is no more common in diabetes.

Vasculitic and purpuric rashes

Vasculitic and purpuric rashes may occur on the feet and shins of patients managed for ulceration of the foot (Figure 8.13).

The cause is not always clear, but the rash may be the result of a drug eruption (allergic response to antibiotics) or a reaction to an infecting organism. Although it may look severe, it settles spontaneously and should be managed with simple cleansing. Figure 8.14 shows purpura which were the result of chronic myeloid leukaemia and thrombocytopenia.

Other skin conditions

Disorders unrelated to diabetes may also occur, such as eczema (Figure 8.15(a)). If the eczematous skin ulcerates, the appearance may resemble that of chronic microvascular ulceration of the skin (Figure 8.15(b)).

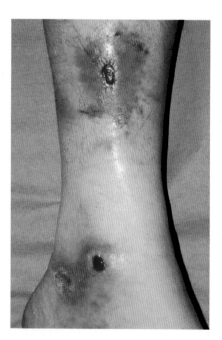

Figure 8.12 The diagnosis of dermatitis artefacta is suggested by the unusual appearance of the lesions, and by the fact that there is usually no sign of any tendency to delayed healing. The integrity of the skin is otherwise well-preserved.

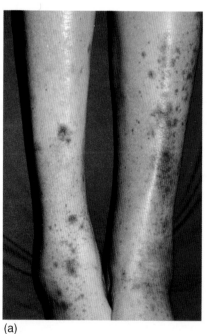

(a)

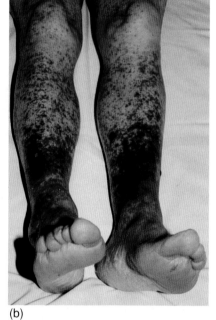

(b)

Figure 8.13(a) A semi-confluent macular rash which is most likely to be the result of a drug reaction. **(b)** A more extensive vasculitic response sometimes occurs while patients are under review for a pre-existing lesion (note the neuropathic ulcer under the second metatarsal head on the left). It is not clear if this is a reaction to any infecting organism or to the drugs which the patients have received.

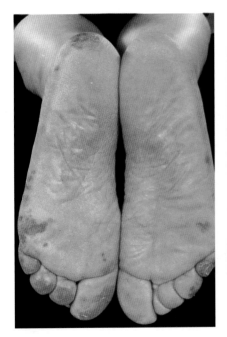

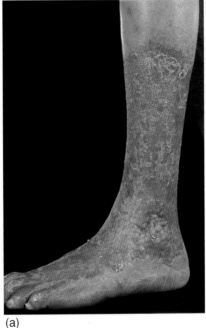

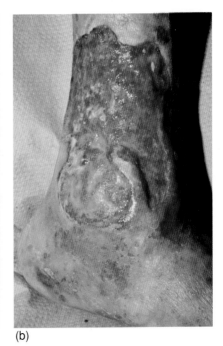

(a)

(b)

Figure 8.14 Purpuric and haemorrhagic lesions on the foot of a man with chronic myeloid leukaemia.

Figure 8.15(a) Ulceration over the lateral malleolus in an area of extensive eczema on the shin of a man with diabetes. **(b)** Microvascular disease can result in chronic, granulating lesions of the shin. These may persist for months or years, but will usually heal with simple, repeated cleansing and dressing. The lesion is very similar in appearance and aetiology to Martorell's ulcer, which is a feature of hypertensive vasculopathy.

MYCOLOGICAL INFECTIONS OF THE FEET AND TOENAILS

People with poorly controlled diabetes are more prone than others to fungal and bacterial infections, and when they have them, they tend to be more severe. Ischaemia may cause nail dystrophy (see Figure 6.14), which allows fungi to penetrate more easily, and resistance to infection is also reduced (Chapter 5). The protective antimicrobial effect of sweat may be lost from a combination of ischaemia and autonomic neuropathy, and changes in the pattern of normal skin flora (Figure 8.16) may permit colonization by pathogenic organisms. Inadequate foot hygiene or increased sweating from socks and tights made of man-made fibres may encourage penetration of fungi.

Tinea pedis

The most frequently encountered mycological infections of the feet are:

1. **dermatophytes** – fungi capable of breaching the epidermal keratin, notably *Trichophyton rubrum*, which is responsible for about 85% of cases;

2. **yeasts** – of which *Candida albicans* is the commonest.

DERMATOPHYTES

Moist, softened, interdigital spaces allow invasion of *Trichophyton rubrum* or *T. interdigitale*, which then

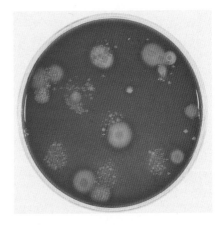

Figure 8.16 Normal bacterial flora which may be cultured from skin (in this case from the unwashed fingertips of schoolchildren). Alteration in this normal flora by, for example, loss of sweating will lead to colonization by others which may behave in a more pathogenic way.

macerate and erode the skin, leaving a fissured area (Figure 8.17).

The characteristic itch will not be felt by someone with peripheral neuropathy, and early infection needs to be sought specifically by regular inspection between the toes. The initial break in the skin allows entry of bacteria. The rate of spread of infection depends on which bacteria have invaded and the degree of ischaemia in the foot.

Fungi can also spread over the surface of the foot; the dyshidrotic form is vesicular and the dry form leaves bare surfaces with epidermal edges (Figure 8.18).

Simple microscopic examination of skin scrapings (taken after swabbing with alcohol) will identify the fungi. If confirmation is required, the skin scales can be cultured.

Treatment is with an antifungal dusting powder or daily topical applications of a cream such as miconazole or ketoconazole, which are active against all common skin fungi, for 2–4 weeks. Careful washing and drying between the toes is important, as is a daily change of socks. Keratolytics such as Whitfield's ointment should not be used.

YEASTS

Candida albicans is most likely to cause paronychia (Figure 8.19), which is inflammation of the tissues surrounding the nail plate.

Maceration, or trauma from, for example, an ingrowing toenail may cause loss of nail cuticle and hence open the seal between the nail fold and the nail plate. This allows colonization by *C. albicans*. The dermis beside the nail becomes swollen, red and painful (except in neuropathy) and secondary bacterial infection occurs. The yeast infection may spread to the nail bed if unchecked (see Onychia, below).

Treatment should be primarily a broad-spectrum antibiotic if there is associated bacterial infection, followed by nystatin, clotrimazole or miconazole creams to suppress the primary infection. Oral ketoconazole can be used in resistant infections, as can terbinafine.

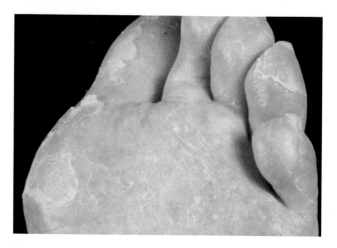

Figure 8.18 The dry form of skin mycosis. This may not respond to topical creams, in which case an oral agent should be used.

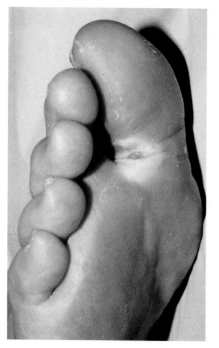

Figure 8.17 (left) Tinea pedis has created a break in the skin which can easily permit secondary bacterial infection.

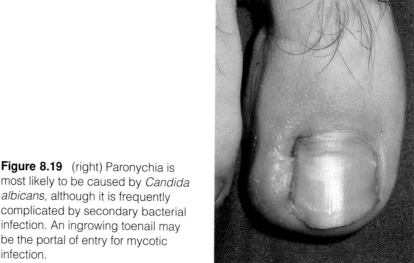

Figure 8.19 (right) Paronychia is most likely to be caused by *Candida albicans*, although it is frequently complicated by secondary bacterial infection. An ingrowing toenail may be the portal of entry for mycotic infection.

Tinea unguium

Onychomycosis of the toenails is almost always caused by *Trichophyton* or *Candida*, which invade the nail plate and nail bed and multiply by metabolizing keratin (Figure 8.20). A definite diagnosis is made by taking nail scrapings if the infection is proximal, or nail clippings (Figure 8.21) if it is distal.

After soaking the clippings in potassium hydroxide for 24 hours, the hyphae can be seen under a microscope. These infestations give rise to a variety of signs.

ONYCHIA

This is inflammation of the nail bed and matrix and is usually associated with prior paronychia. The initial break may have been caused by a traumatic incident, but is often the result of candidiasis. Bacterial infection then causes oedema and suppuration, with separation of the nail from its bed and discolouration. Drainage of any pus will relieve pressure and pain and the treatment is the same as for paronychia.

ONYCHOLYSIS

This term refers variously to flaking of the nail or to detachment from the nail bed. The invading fungus disorganizes the structure of the nail, which then lifts from its bed, starting either at the edges or at the distal end (Figure 8.22). Air enters into pockets created beneath the nail and this makes it look white. If they become filled with dirt, the nail is discoloured.

ONYCHAUXIS AND ONYCHOGRYPHOSIS

The fungal infections often cause thickening of the nail by excessive horn production from beneath, although it can occasionally be caused by trauma. The nail plate then becomes difficult to cut. In

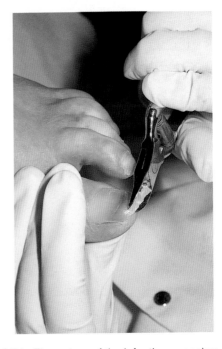

Figure 8.21 The nature of the infecting organism can be defined by microscopic examination of nails clippings.

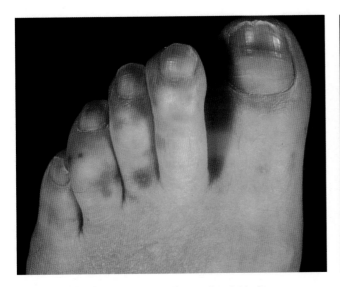

Figure 8.20 Tinea unguium. The nails of this foot are discoloured by infection by either dermatophytes (*Trichophyton* spp.) or yeasts (*Candida albicans*). The red mottling of the skin is caused by chilblains.

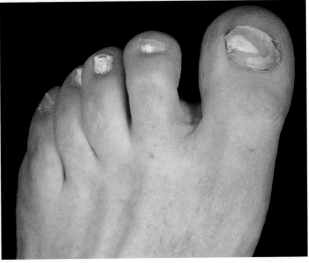

Figure 8.22 White patches appear on the nail where it is lifted up from its bed as a result of infection with *T. rubrum*.

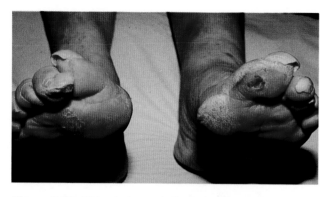

Figure 8.23 This photograph illustrates three abnormalities: (1) there is gross deformity of the nails from onychogryphosis; (2) psoriasis is causing exaggerated callus formation around the edges of the foot; (3) peripheral neuropathy is causing callus under the second metatarsal head on the right and the ulcer on the hallux on the left. Of the three it is the first which will be most obvious on casual inspection, but the third which poses the greatest risk to the foot.

onychogryphosis (Figure 8.23) the nail is thickened so that it becomes like a horn.

Such hypertrophic nails eventually become spongy and start to disintegrate, or they may be accidentally torn off. Regular chiropody is essential, because the person will be unable to cut the nails him/herself. It should be noted, however, that nails will only become hypertrophic if they have a good blood supply, and this means that the foot with onychogryphosis cannot be ischaemic. It may look awful but it is not at particular risk.

MANAGEMENT OF ONYCHOMYCOSIS (NAIL INFECTION)

The problem associated with treating nail mycoses is that nails grow slowly and treatment is required for 2–6 months. Systemic therapy against dermatophytes with griseofulvin has now been largely superseded by terbinafine.

9 Chiropody

Chiropodists are those members of the multidisciplinary team who provide regular, routine foot care. For this reason they are often the first to notice potential problems (Figure 9.1), to detect ulcers that have occurred as a consequence of unnoticed trauma, and to observe when an ulcer has become infected.

Those who work in the community may be the first to suspect undiagnosed diabetes mellitus when a patient presents with a suggestive lesion. Consequently they should work in close contact with other health care professionals in order to alert them to the need for further action.

The chiropodist is also in an ideal position to teach the patient about the relationship between diabetes and foot problems, emphasizing the need for regular inspection and a sensible approach to hygiene (Figure 9.2).

Thus they can give general advice on washing, changing clothes regularly and drying between the toes – in order to prevent the accumulation of moist detritus in the toe webs or in the cracks beneath the toes, which provides an excellent climate for fungal invasion.

SKIN CARE

The feet are often dry and scaly as a result of anhidrosis, which is itself secondary to autonomic neuropathy (Chapter 7). Regular application of a moisturising cream will help soften the skin and, hopefully, prevent the development of skin fissures – which may be painful (Figure 9.3), and which may

also become secondarily infected. When deep fissuring has occurred, silver nitrate solution can be used to cauterize the edges of the crack, followed by hydrocortisone cream.

NAIL CARE

Obesity or poor eyesight may prevent people cutting their nails or, if they do attempt it, they may cut the surrounding skin or leave a portion of a nail uncut, which could cause trauma to a neighbouring toe. Inexpert cutting may also result in an ingrowing toenail, which is sometimes thought to start with a

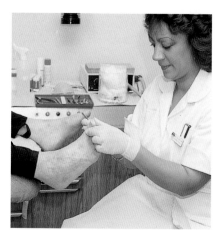

Figure 9.2 While working on the feet, all chiropodists take the opportunity to emphasize to the patient the need for proper foot care.

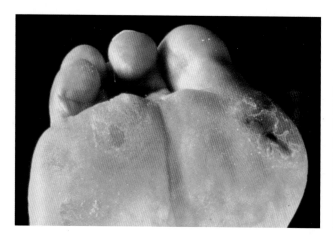

Figure 9.1 This foot is seriously at risk from the combination of deformity and lack of chiropody. A chiropodist would note that haemorrhage had occurred within the area of callus over the first metatarsal head and would predict that ulceration was imminent.

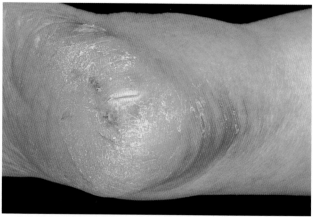

Figure 9.3 Fissuring around the heel may be prevented by use of emollient creams.

splinter of nail penetrating the surrounding tissue, causing infection and inflammation (Figure 9.4).

Toenails should therefore be cut short, but not too short; and there should be no remaining sharp edges. The services of state-registered chiropodists are essential for providing such routine care to the nails of the more elderly and infirm.

Mycological infection of nails causes thickened nails with increased curvature, sometimes leading to partial detachment from the nail bed (Figure 9.5); this has been dealt with in greater detail in Chapter 8.

If left unattended, they will create extra pressure from shoes and may also be accidentally torn off. Mycotic nails are difficult to cut with ordinary clip-

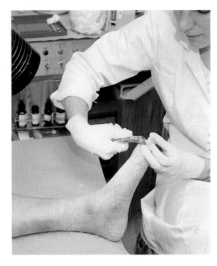

Figure 9.6 It can be impossible to cut thickened and dystrophic nails without the help of a chiropodist.

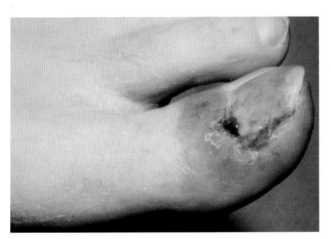

Figure 9.4 Careless nail clipping may leave a sharp spike, which may then grow into the adjacent soft tissue and allow secondary bacterial infection.

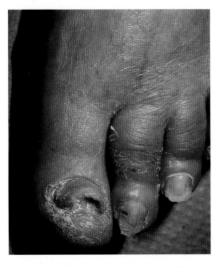

Figure 9.5 Mycological infection of the nail on the hallux has caused it to thicken, curl and lift from its base. The other nails are long and may damage the skin of adjacent toes. This foot needs expert care.

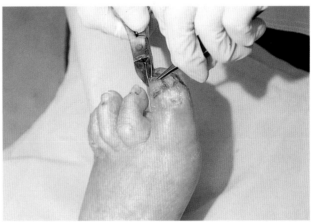

Figure 9.7 Removal of the nail may be necessary in the management of mycological infection, to permit drainage of subungual infection or to reduce the risk of trauma to adjacent toes.

pers and scissors and should be regularly trimmed by a chiropodist (Figure 9.6) in order to keep them thin and short.

If the chances of accidental trauma to a nail are high, if subungual haematomas occur (which is a sign that the foot is anaesthetic from peripheral neuropathy), or if for any other reason it is felt that more aggressive treatment is indicated, then either antimycotic therapy or nail avulsion should be considered (Figure 9.7). Nail eradication with phenol alcohol is a third option, but should not be undertaken if the blood supply to the foot is compromised.

CALLOSITIES

The development of plantar callus is usually the result of redistribution of weight on the sole of the foot as a consequence of motor neuropathy (Chapter 7). Callus on the dorsal and lateral aspects of the foot may be the result of deformities such as bunions (Figure 9.8), or unnoticed pressure from shoes (particularly new ones) rubbing.

The inflammatory response of soft tissue to constant shearing forces or continual pressure is to form a protective callus by increasing keratin production. If left untreated, this becomes harder and creates a protrusion on the surface of the foot, which in turn creates more pressure and necrosis beneath. If this leads to ulceration of the skin, the wound may become infected and this may be the first time the

patient notices that anything is wrong. The task of the chiropodist is to prevent excessive build-up of callus by regular debridement with a scalpel (Figure 9.9).

Corns

Hard corns (from the Latin *cornu* = horn) may be the consequence of toe deformities or shoes which are too tight, or both. They occur characteristically on the dorsal interphalangeal joints (Figure 9.10) or on the plantar surface beneath the metatarsal heads, but they may be found interdigitally or subungually.

A corn is an area of callus which has evolved a central plug of hard skin due to continued lateral pressure. Corn plasters, which contain salicylic acid that softens keratinized cells, should not be used in diabetes because damage to the surrounding skin may cause ulceration which may then be slow to heal.

ULCERS

Neuropathic ulcers

The classic neuropathic ulcer has a deep, clean centre enclosed by hyperkeratotic callus. The surrounding callus must be kept to a minimum by regular chiropody, and any necrotic or infected tissue must

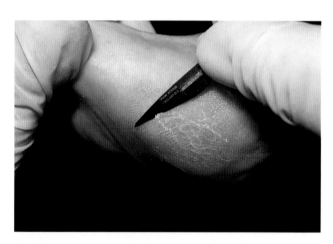

Figure 9.8 Sharp debridement of callus which has formed over the medial aspect of the first metatarsophalangeal joint, as well as elsewhere on the toes.

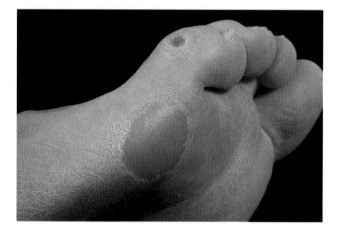

Figure 9.9 Regular and effective control of callus accumulation will prevent the build-up of pressure sufficient to cause ulceration.

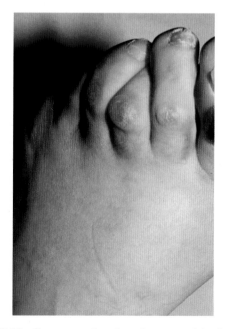

Figure 9.10 Corns over the dorsal aspect of the interphalangeal joints have developed because of pressure from shoes that are not deep enough to accommodate the foot.

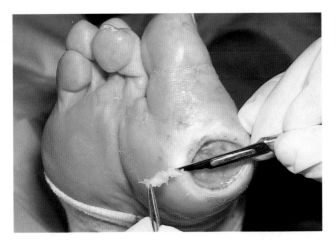

Figure 9.11 Paring of callus around the rim of a neuropathic ulcer helps healing to occur from the edge.

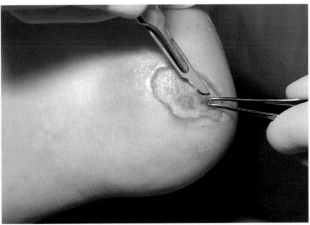

Figure 9.12 Piecemeal debridement of slough is necessary because the wound must be clean before it will heal.

also be pared away to leave only healthy tissue. This promotes granulation from the base of the ulcer and epithelialization from the rim (Figure 9.11).

Neuroischaemic ulcers

Callus is usually absent from the ischaemic foot, but debridement may be necessary to remove slough (Figure 9.12).

Amputation sites

The purpose of debridement is to create the best possible environment for wound healing. Healing will be helped if a postoperative wound is kept clean (Figure 9.13). Ray amputations may tend to accumulate callus around the edges of the wound, and these need to be trimmed.

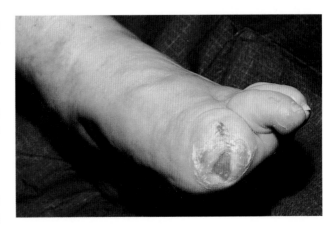

Figure 9.13 Callus may well accumulate around the base of an amputated digit and, as for neuropathic ulceration of the sole (Figure 9.11), must be pared away to allow epithelialization to occur.

THE PLACE OF CHIROPODY IN ULCER MANAGEMENT

The place of chiropody is central to good ulcer management, and it is unfortunate that many chiropodists work in relative isolation from other health care professionals, both in the community and in hospitals. Not only is chiropody an essential adjunct to overall wound care, it is in many cases the only treatment which is given. In those in whom more definitive treatment is impossible because their general health prohibits general anaesthesia, chiropody may keep the foot usable and prevent the loss of the limb from spreading infection (Figure 9.14). Patient, repeated cleaning and debridement may lead to healing of very extensive areas of ulceration (Figure 9.15).

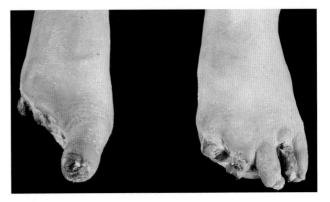

Figure 9.14 This man was unable to have definitive treatment for his progressively gangrenous toes because a recent severe myocardial infarction made him unfit for general anaesthesia. However, repeated careful cleansing and debridement (and treatment of occasional intercurrent infection) enabled him to keep both his feet until he died peacefully, in his sleep, 2 years later.

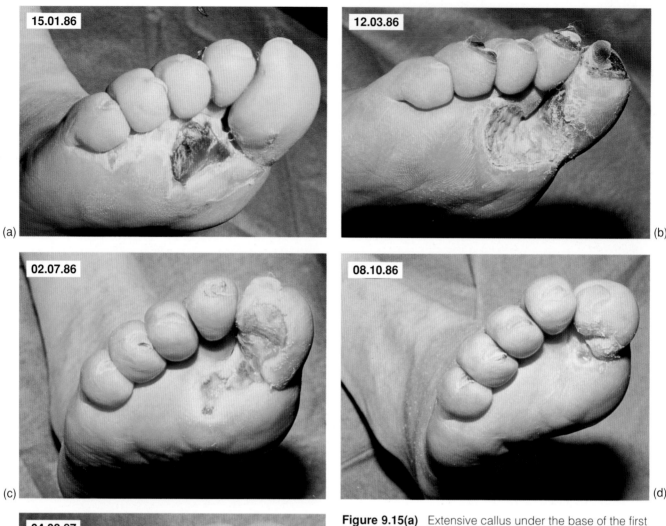

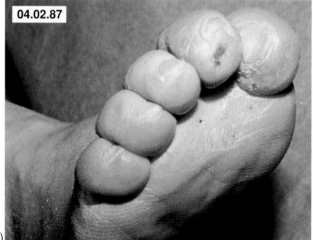

Figure 9.15(a) Extensive callus under the base of the first three toes with a blood blister indicating the start of critical ischaemic necrosis beneath it. **(b)** Removal of callus has revealed an indolent, pasty-looking ulcer which shows little signs of early healing. New blood blisters have developed at the ends of three toes. **(c)** After a further 4 months of patient, repeated treatment, the ulcerated area is starting to close in from the outside. **(d)** The ulcer has almost completely healed. **(e)** Complete healing has been achieved, but note that the hallux has now been pulled down by scar tissue and this has led to secondary neuropathic ulceration of the tip of the second toe. This settled quickly in response to conventional management, but it emphasizes the need to provide fitted footwear as quickly as possible after a mainly neuropathic lesion has been treated.

10   Applications and dressings

Successful management of foot ulcers requires an understanding of all the processes which caused them in the first place and those that contribute to their continuation. Part of this involves providing the exposed tissues with the best environment possible for healing to take place – in other words, cleaning and dressing them properly. Proper management of the surface of the wound is, therefore, a critical aspect of care – even if there is sometimes a tendency for people to think that it is the only one.

Nevertheless, superficial wound management is not always well done. Few doctors and nurses have been taught to select logically from the large number of applications available for cleaning and treating the wound, and from the wide choice of dressings. They tend to rely more on habit, cost and convenience.

Moreover, the possible harmful effects of dressing wounds are not always recognized – an inappropriate choice of method may sometimes delay healing.

THE HEALING PROCESS

Ulcers are associated with an area of skin loss and hence heal by secondary intention. Normal healing (Figure 10.1) is characterized by the following sequence:

1. arrest of haemorrhage, with the area being sealed by blood clot;
2. inflammation, with invasion of the area by

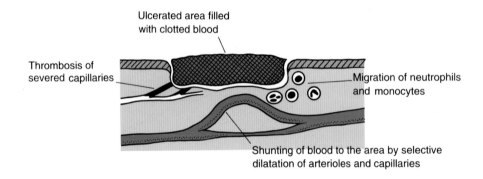

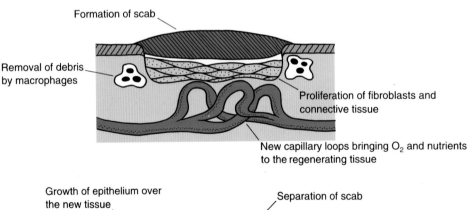

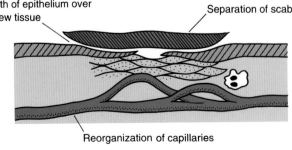

Figure 10.1 The process of normal healing.

neutrophils and monocytes; blood clot and dried inflammatory exudate combine to form a hard scab which isolates the wound from the exterior;
3. growth of new capillaries;
4. proliferation of fibroblasts and connective tissue, collagen and extracellular matrix;
5. epithelialization, with new epithelium growing from the edge to cover the exposed area;
6. organization of scar tissue.

Since the greatest risk to the healing of healthy tissue is infection, the formation of the scab is crucial (Figure 10.2). It forms an impermeable barrier to the outside, while any bacteria and debris which are present beneath it are eliminated by macrophages (Figure 10.3). The scab also preserves the microenvironment of the healing tissue, protecting it from cold and from drying out – the healing process continues most rapidly if the cells involved are kept warm and moist.

Healing of ulcers in diabetes

The problem with diabetes is that the healing process is not normal (Figure 10.4).

The blood supply may be impaired through macrovascular disease and the capillaries may function abnormally because of microvascular disease. Thus the inflammatory process is reduced and

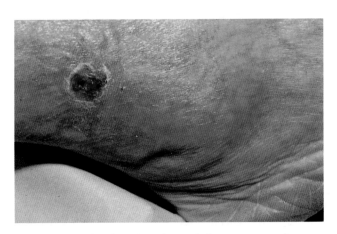

Figure 10.2 The function of a scab is to preserve the microenvironment of the regenerating tissue.

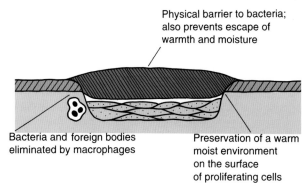

Figure 10.3 This drawing illustrates the different protective functions of a healthy scab.

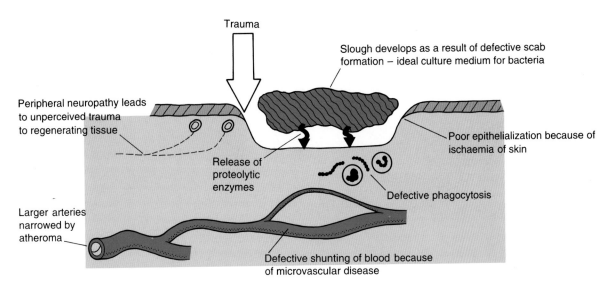

Figure 10.4 Defective wound healing in diabetes.

delayed, with defective formation of scab and defective delivery of neutrophils and macrophages. For these reasons the wound is particularly prone to invasion by pathogenic organisms and, once infection occurs, it will delay healing further. Such infection is especially likely because the phagocytic action of neutrophils and macrophages is reduced in diabetes. Furthermore, the person with an ulcer may be unaware of it for some time because sensation in the foot is reduced by peripheral neuropathy, and by continuing to walk on it they destroy any new tissue which forms, as well as increasing the likelihood of infection.

For these reasons, ulcers which occur in diabetes must be identified as quickly as possible and dressed effectively; the dressings should act as an artificial scab.

SLOUGH AND ESCHAR

Slough is a mass of necrotic cells, exudate, foreign material and bacteria (Figure 10.5).

It develops as a result of defective scab formation which is the consequence of the multiple functional defects of diabetes listed above. Once slough forms it acts as a medium for the proliferation of bacteria. These release proteolytic enzymes which inhibit wound healing. When slough is black on the surface, it is called **eschar**. Eschar may be either soft or hard.

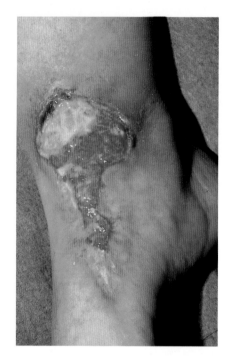

Figure 10.5 This wound is healing at the lower end where it is clean and more free from slough. The slough at the upper end acts as a medium for the proliferation of bacteria which release proteolytic enzymes and inhibit the healing process.

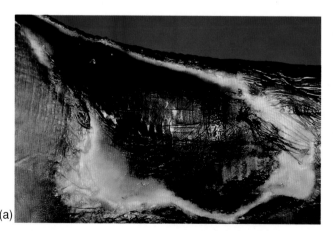

(a)

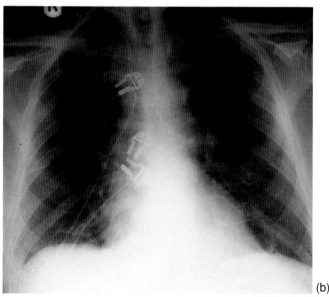

(b)

Figure 10.6(a) This lady was frail, blind and had bad heart failure. She burnt her shin on a hot water bottle. When a consultant surgeon advised amputation, she sensibly refused. She kept her leg and died peacefully of her heart disease 6 months later. **(b)** The patient's chest X-ray, showing signs of heart failure.

PRINCIPLES OF WOUND MANAGEMENT

There are two broad aspects of management of an ulcer on the foot of a diabetic:

1. promotion of healing in those in whom there is a chance it will occur;
2. simple prevention of further complications in those in whom the chance of healing is minimal.

It is important for this distinction to be made because the choice of wound care is dependent on it. Thus, it may be recognized that an extensive wound in a person made frail by, for example, ischaemic heart disease (Figure 10.6) will never heal and if so, the attempt should be to keep it dry and free from secondary infection.

The same is true of the large scabs that may develop as the result of pressure on the heel of a person immobilized by illness (Figure 10.7): they are often best left alone – provided they are dry and uninfected. Since healing is never likely to occur, the object is not to promote healing but to prevent complications.

Thus, the first aspect of wound management is to define its aim and once it is defined, it needs to be clearly stated so that all the different people involved in care are aware of it. The other aspects are:

1. debridement;
2. cleaning;
3. applications;
4. dressings.

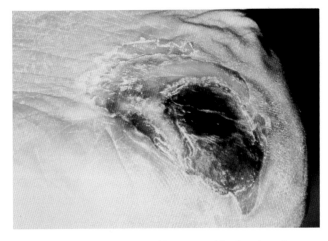

Figure 10.7 When a wound is covered by hard eschar, there are two options: to remove it or to leave it in place. If it is incomplete or starting to lift, as shown here, it is better removed to allow more effective cleaning of the tissue below. If it completely covers the ulcer, however, and if there is no sign of moistness around the edge, then it is sometimes best left in place.

Debridement of slough and eschar

Slough and soft eschar must be removed in order to prevent secondary infection and to promote healing of the healthy tissues beneath. Note, however, that hardened eschar acts as an impenetrable barrier to bacteria and to moisture, and if it extends to the edges of the wound it may serve as a secondary scab (Figure 10.7). In such cases it is often best left in place

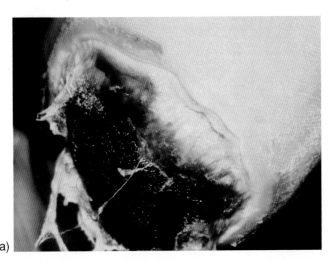

(a)

Figure 10.8(a) Wet slough must be removed because the wound will never heal and spreading secondary infection is inevitable. Extensive involvement of the heel poses a special problem because the soft tissue of the heel pad will not regenerate once it has been destroyed.

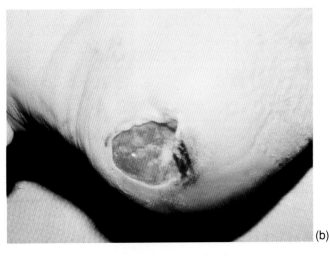

(b)

(b) Although 50% of heel ulcers never heal, success can be had from patient, repeated debridement – which needs to be continued over many months. This shows the same heel as in **(a)** after a period of 5 months.

because it may be sealing the ulcer better than any dressing will do.

Effective removal of slough can lead to healing of even the worst looking ulcers (Figure 10.8). There are two approaches: sharp (surgical) and gentle (chemical or osmotic).

SHARP DEBRIDEMENT

It may be necessary to debride the area under general anaesthesia – with the objective of removing all necrotic matter at once and leaving only healthy bleeding tissue at the edges of the wound. All too often, however, the person is unfit for elective general anaesthesia and the aim is then to remove the dead tissue progressively at each dressing. Such piecemeal debridement is undertaken with scalpel and forceps (Figure 10.9).

GENTLE DEBRIDEMENT

Moist material can be removed at dressing with a saline moistened swab, or by saline irrigation. Persistent gentle debridement can lead to healing of extensive areas of ulceration (Figure 10.10).

The process of physically removing the dead tissue

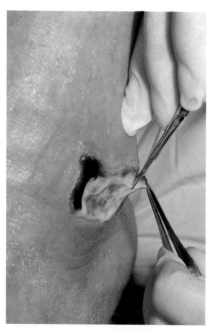

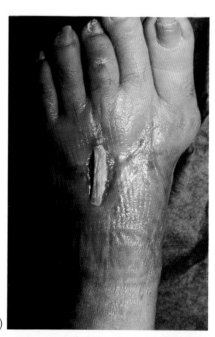

Figure 10.9 (left) Piecemeal physical debridement of surface slough.

Figure 10.10(a) This wound shows signs of active healing although the exposed tendon has to be sacrificed to permit the skin to close over. **(b)** The development of healthy granulation tissue is followed by the spread of epithelium from the edges of the wound. **(c)** Almost complete healing. **(d)** Complete healing has been achieved but the removal of the extensor tendon has resulted in plantar flexion of the toe. This toe is now particularly liable to develop neuropathic ulceration over the knuckle or the tip, and the provision of fitted footwear should be seriously considered. (a)

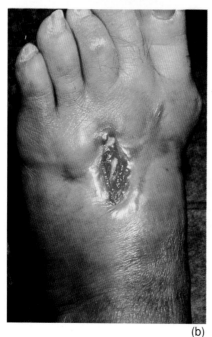

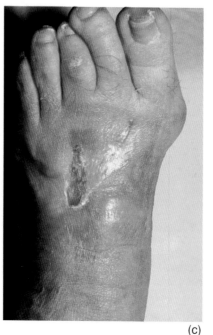

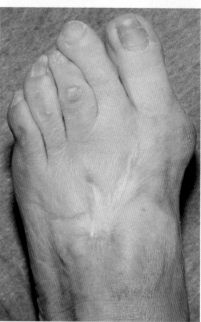

(b)   (c)   (d)

can also be helped by the use of various applications. Such 'desloughing agents' work either by softening the slough to make it easier to wash off or osmotically by drying it so that it adheres to the application and can be removed with it when the dressing is changed.

DESLOUGHING AGENTS

Weak acids

A number of applications are based on the debriding effect of weak acids. Aserbine is a mixture of malic, benzoic and salicylic acids and 5% acetic acid can also be used. These preparations are cheap and often effective (Figure 10.11).

The active principle of Variclene is lactic acid, but it is eight times more expensive than Aserbine. Comparative costs of these preparations are listed in Table 10.1.

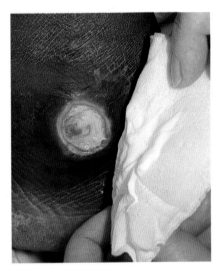

Figure 10.11 Application of Aserbine to a moist wound. The combination of weak acids helps to break down slough.

Table 10.1 Approximate costs of some applications and dressings (1994 prices)

		Cost (£)	Amount
Debriding agents			
Weak acids	Aserbine	1.40	100 g
	Variclene	5.50	50 g
Gels/colloids	Debrisan paste	6.00	10 g
	Iodosorb beads	2.30	3 g
	Intrasite gel	2.10	15 g
	* Geliperm paste	4.00	20 g
	* Granuflex paste	4.00	30 g
	Granuflex wafers	2.50	10 × 10 cm
Enzymatic	Varidase	9.00	1 vial
Alginates	* Kaltostat rope	3.50	2 g
	Kaltostat sheets	1.80	7.5 × 12 cm
	Sorbsan sheets	1.80	10 × 10 cm
Cleaning agents	Saline	0.10	25 ml
	Betadine	2.00	500 ml
	0.05% chlorhexidine	0.10	25 ml
	Potassium permanganate	0.05	4 l
	Hioxyl cream	1.75	25 g
Dressings	Melolin	0.25	10 × 10 cm
	Paraffin gauze	0.30	10 × 10 cm
	Opsite	1.30	10 × 12 cm
	Granuflex sheets	2.00	10 × 10 cm
	* Allevyn	2.00	10 × 10 cm

* Not available on the NHS Drug Tariff

Hydrogen peroxide

While unmodified hydrogen peroxide is probably active for only a few minutes after being applied, it may last for up to 8 hours when stabilized in a cream.

Enzyme preparations

The rationale for the use of enzyme preparations is that the enzymes digest the slough (and, presumably, other tissue as well). They are expensive and have to be made up freshly each time they are applied. Varidase contains streptokinase and there is a theoretical risk of hypersensitivity from antibody formation in those who have previously had thrombolytic therapy.

Gels, colloids and polymer beads

All act osmotically by adsorbing necrotic material into their matrix. They can be left for 2–3 days to allow maximal adsorption but very wet wounds need to be redressed more frequently (Figure 10.12).

At redressing, the matrix and absorbed material is washed off with saline. Gels appear to be equally effective although Geliperm comes in a variety of formulations – in sheets for shallow ulcers and granules for deep ones.

Colloids come in a variety of forms, including pastes, and wafers for packing deeper wounds. They are available as impregnated semi-occlusive dressings. The action of colloids is similar to the gels but they are designed to be left in place for longer (Figure 10.13).

However, prolonged occlusion may lead to maceration of healthy tissue and may encourage the proliferation of bacteria trapped when dressing takes place – especially in wetter wounds.

Osmotic starch–polymer beads are cheap and particularly useful for removing slough in deeper wounds, even though they sometimes become quite hard and difficult to remove. Iodosorb acts on a similar principle, but the granules are impregnated with iodine which may help to reduce infection. It is possible that sugar paste and granular honey (which are used in some centres) are just as effective osmotic agents as those above, and cheaper – even though the dressings need to be changed at least once or twice a day, and so the true cost is higher than it seems (Table 10.2). The approximate costs of different dressings and applications are listed in Table 10.1.

Table 10.2 Formulation for sugar pastes used at Northwick Park Hospital

	Thin paste	Thick paste
Castor sugar	1200 g	1200 g
Icing sugar (no additives)	1800 g	1800 g
Polyethylene glycol	1416 ml	686 ml
Hydrogen peroxide	23.1 ml	19 ml

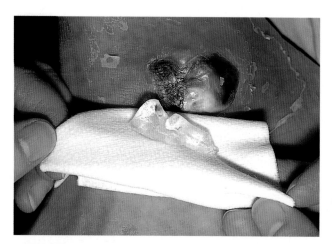

Figure 10.12 Hygroscopic gels and other polymers, beads and starches are all effective as desloughing agents. Sloughy tissue becomes adherent to the dressing material and is removed with it when the dressing is changed. They are particularly suitable for deep and irregular wounds because they prevent accumulation of exudate in crevices.

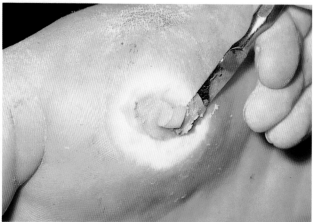

Figure 10.13 Deep wounds can be filled with colloid preparations which are available as pastes and beads.

Cleaning

Once obvious slough is removed, the objective of cleaning a wound is the removal of microscopic foreign bodies and potentially pathogenic bacteria. It is not necessary to keep the whole wound surface completely sterile and the chances are that attempts to eliminate all bacteria increase the risk of colonization by pathogenic ones.

Cleaning should be gentle; vigorous scrubbing will destroy regenerating tissue, as will the use of more powerful antiseptics (Figure 10.14).

Sterile saline is probably adequate for most purposes, although the use of a mild antiseptic such as 0.05% chlorhexidine may prevent help to prevent reinfection between dressings. Such solutions should be kept at room temperature, and not in a refrigerator; if they are cold when applied, they will slow the metabolism of regenerating cells. Povidone-iodine is also widely used but there is evidence that it may sometimes delay healing – povidone-iodine spray may cause unwanted drying of the surface of the wound and leave particulate foreign bodies which may slow the process of regeneration. Weak acid preparations such as 5% acetic acid may also be considered, and 0.01% potassium permanganate is especially useful if the surrounding skin is excoriated or delicate – even though it stains it brown.

BATHING THE ULCER BEFORE DRESSING

A useful prelude is to soak the foot in a basin of salt water (two dessertspoonfuls of table salt in a washing-up bowl of lukewarm water). It should not be done for more than 5 minutes, however, because it may make the surrounding healthy skin soggy. Soaking helps to soften the dressing and eases the removal of particulate foreign matter when the wound is later cleansed. Some people use a dilute solution of povidone-iodine in place of saline (Figure 10.15).

It also helps if the patient keeps the whole area as clean as possible. All too often, patients are told not to get the wound wet by putting the foot in the bath. This illogical advice does nothing but worsen the accumulation of filth (Figure 10.16) on the affected leg, and makes the patient miserable because s/he is denied a bath for weeks on end.

Applications

TOPICAL ANTIBIOTICS

In general, there is no place for the use of topical antibiotics. If the foot is infected, antibiotics should be given systemically. The only exceptions to this are

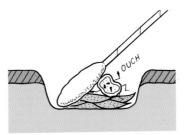
Vigorous scrubbing will destroy superficial layers of regenerating cells

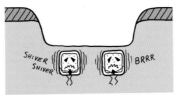
Prolonged exposure to the air may cause desiccation and cooling of surface cells

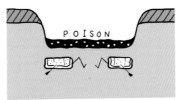
Potent antiseptics will affect host tissue as well

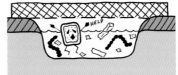
Failure to pack a deep wound will lead to accumulation of exudate which becomes secondarily infected

Figure 10.14 Cleaning wounds may sometimes have a detrimental effect on healing tissue.

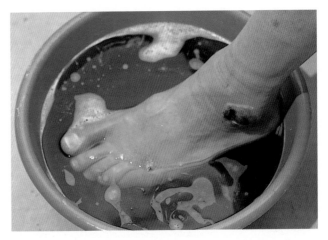

Figure 10.15 Soaking of the foot – for no more than 5 minutes – in lukewarm salt water or very dilute antiseptic helps the subsequent removal of hardened dressings and of slough. It also ensures that the whole foot is kept clean.

the use of antifungal agents for tinea, and metronidazole gel – which is said to reduce the smell caused by superficial infection with anaerobic bacteria. Silver sulphadiazine cream (Flamazine) confers no particular advantages – even though it sometimes seems to work as an effective desloughing agent.

APPLICATIONS WHICH PROMOTE HEALING

Alginates

It is possible that alginate preparations (derived from seaweed) help regenerating tissue by filling the wound with a scaffolding of natural fibres, and there is experimental evidence to suggest that they promote growth of connective tissue. They are particularly useful for packing deeper wet wounds, and for eliminating the accumulation of unwanted exudate (Figure 10.17).

However, they are inappropriate for ulcers with only minimal exudate because they may dry the surface too much. This dehydration can be reduced by soaking the dressing in saline before applying it.

Growth factors

In the near future it is probable that a new range of applications will become available that actively promote the growth of connective tissue. Initial trials with preparations containing growth factors, such as platelet-derived growth factor (PDGF), are encouraging.

Applications to promote epithelialization

Some wounds develop healthy granulation tissue but are slow to cover it with new epithelium, presumably because of relative ischaemia of the skin. Repeated sharp debridement of the edge helps – probably by enabling more effective cleansing of the edge of the wound (Figure 10.18). Colloid dressings are also thought to encourage epithelialization.

Occasionally, the granulation tissue may become exuberant and heaped-up (Figure 10.19) and this may itself impede its being covered by epidermis. In such cases the extent of granulation can be reduced by applying 1% hydrocortisone cream (sometimes combined with the topical antibiotic, neomycin), and this may help.

Skin grafting

If epithelialization is delayed, skin grafting may work well – provided the wound is shallow and its base is formed by healthy granulation tissue.

Dressings

The purpose of a dressing is to protect the wound from infection and to preserve the optimal microenvironment for regenerating tissue. Thus, the dressing needs to:

1. be impermeable to bacteria;
2. insulate the wound from cold air and incidental trauma;

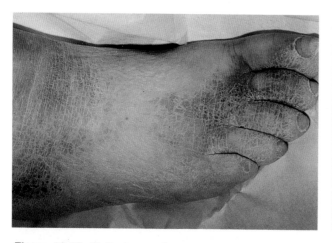

Figure 10.16 Patients are often told that they must keep the affected foot dry and that they must not have a bath or shower until it is healed. There is no basis for this and all it does is to make the foot dirty and the patient uncomfortable.

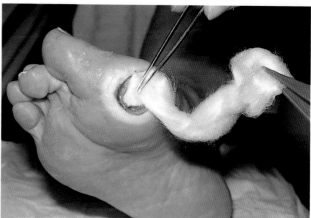

Figure 10.17 Packing of a deep clean wound with alginate rope. The alginate helps prevent accumulation of exudate and is also said to act as a scaffold for regenerating cells. If the wound is moist, it can be packed with dry rope. If it is not so moist, the rope should be soaked in saline before being applied.

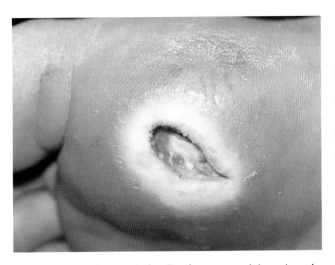

Figure 10.18 Removal of callus from around the edge of a neuropathic ulcer will encourage healing. Different authorities have different views on how aggressive such debridement should be. Some suggest that avascular callus should be pared away until the surrounding skin starts to bleed.

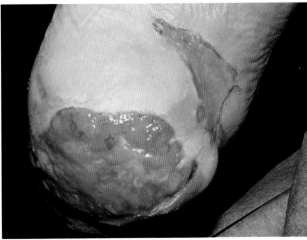

Figure 10.19 The reason for accumulation of excessive granulation tissue is not known, but it presumably indicates that healing of connective tissue continues while epithelialization is delayed. When the granulation tissue is proud and heaped-up, as shown here, it may itself inhibit the closure of the wound. Hydrocortisone cream is effective at suppressing it.

3. preserve a layer of moisture over the regenerating tissue – thin enough to prevent the cells from becoming dehydrated, but not so much that the risk of infection is increased;
4. be non-adherent – such that the surface areas of the wound are not torn off when it is redressed;
5. be socially acceptable by hiding the wound and eliminating odour.

If these requirements are satisfied, it follows that the dressing should be as cheap and as convenient to apply as possible. Dressings which are designed to be retained in place are obviously more desirable than those which have to be changed daily, but there is a danger that a wound that is covered and not cleaned for several days will become either macerated or infected.

CONVENTIONAL GAUZE

Cotton gauze dressings have a limited place because they are not impermeable to bacteria (especially when damp). Moreover they adhere to the wound surface and harden when they dry. Occasionally, however, they are used in order to dry an area of extensive slough, because effective drying will destroy bacteria and may promote the secondary development of a scab. Sometimes this is the best policy for an area of wet necrosis in someone whose overall prognosis is obviously poor for other reasons

and in whom it may be the best way of preventing spreading tissue infection. In these circumstances there is also a place for using povidone-iodine dry powder. A similar approach is useful in trying to dry the edge of any demarcated area of gangrene – such as the sloughy base of a single black toe which is not thought suitable for surgery.

PARAFFIN TULLE

Tulle dressings offer better insulation of the healing tissue and are also non-adherent and easy to remove (Figure 10.20).

They require a surface dressing but are cheap and non-toxic and have a particular place in the management of clean superficial lesions which are on the verge of epithelializing. Dressings that contain an antibiotic preparation have no apparent advantages.

OTHER LOW-ADHERENT DRESSINGS

The absorbent part of some dressings have a non-adherent coating which is applied to the wound. Other non-adherent sheets are rather more absorbent and hence better for wetter ulcers but require an additional surface dressing.

HYDROCOLLOID DRESSINGS

Colloid-impregnated dressings are particularly useful for superficial wounds with light to moderate

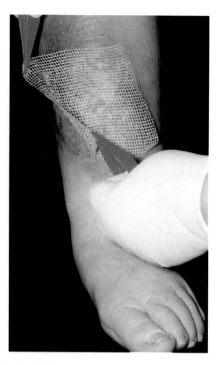

Figure 10.20 When the wound is superficial and clean, it is important to make sure that the process of cleaning and dressing it does not do damage to the regenerating tissue. The use of paraffin gauze prevents the dressing from becoming adherent to the wound.

exudate. The colloid absorbs the exudate. Although possibly no more effective overall than simpler preparations, they are designed to be left in place for several days and are therefore cheaper and more convenient. Infrequent dressing will also cause less disturbance to the newly forming tissue, but may cause maceration of surrounding normal skin.

SEMI-PERMEABLE FILM

Synthetic film sheets are available which are permeable to water and to air (unless the pores become blocked by exudate) and are used by some to insulate wounds. They often seem to be left in place too long and cause maceration. A macerated wound is liable to secondary infection.

ACTIVATED CHARCOAL

Dressings impregnated with activated charcoal are said to reduce smell from surface infection.

Compression bandaging

Compression bandaging is widely used in clinical circumstances to promote wound healing by reducing the accumulation of exudate in the wound, as well as limiting oedema of surrounding tissues. Its place in the management of diabetic foot ulcers is limited, however, because it may compromise a blood supply which is already parlous.

Alleviation of pressure

Walking induces injury to the surface of the wound and also increases the nutrient requirements of the tissues of the foot, and it follows that the ulcerated area should be rested as much as possible. Maximum rest is important in the early stages, especially if the wound is complicated by surrounding infection. However, the overall healing time of diabetic ulcers is so long that it is impractical for a person to rest the foot completely. To ask them to do so is unfair: they are unlikely to comply and if they do, they may become much weakened and depressed by enforced confinement. It is better to urge them to rest the foot 'as much as possible', and to adopt other measures to spread the weight from the ulcerated area. These include the use of slippers, soft shoes, pillows, footstools, protection pads, Scotchcast boots and the like.

Psychological and social aspects of wound management

Certain behavioural factors – of both the patient and the professional – contribute to decisions concerning management. Many stem from the unpleasantness of the underlying condition, which is perceived by patient and carers alike. It is possible that this is one reason why many doctors tend to leave management to nurses, their only contribution being to sign prescriptions. On the other hand nurses may feel uncertain about optimum management and unsure about where to seek advice. They may tend to favour only those applications which they have used before.

Other subtle factors may condition the choice of certain preparations. Thus, a desire to sterilize the area may lead to a preference for brightly coloured preparations: if a wound is stained brown or bright green, it helps to emphasize that it has been effectively cleaned. Similarly, an attempt to insulate the cleaned wound from all risk of infection leads to the possibly inappropriate use of plastic film dressings and the certainly inappropriate ban on having a bath.

Finally, the ever-present squeeze on resources leads professionals to choose the dressings that require to be done least often. For those ulcers which are sloughy or wet this is usually unwise and may contribute to the development of secondary infection.

Potentially adverse effects of dressings

Healing can sometimes be hampered by the dressing process as much as helped by it. Vigorous scrubbing of the surface may destroy the regenerating layer of cells while surface cooling and drying will also cause temporary inhibition of their metabolism. The use of powerful antiseptics may also harm the normal cells as much as invading bacteria and dry powder sprays are usually unwise because of the drying they cause. Debriding agents may sometimes irritate the surrounding skin. Occlusive dressings that are left in place too long on wet wounds may lead to an accumulation of exudate, which often becomes secondarily infected.

SUMMARY

In order to help heal a wound it must be debrided, cleaned and dressed on a regular basis. Debridement is designed to uncover healthy tissue and to free it from a coating of dead cells and exudate which harbours bacteria. Cleaning should be efficient but gentle and may or may not be followed by the application of specific preparations. These preparations have several functions: continued chemical removal of slough; packing of a deep wound in order to absorb excessive exudate; and, potentially, direct promotion of cell proliferation and wound healing. The dressing is designed to act as an artificial scab, to protect the microenvironment of the wound and to insulate it from physical trauma. The process needs to be repeated as often as is necessary to remove dead tissue from the surface and to prevent its reaccumulation. A suggested approach is summarized in Table 10.3, and some preparations are listed in Table 10.4.

Table 10.3 Suggestions for management of different types of foot ulcer

1.	Shallow, clean, no exudate	
	Cleaning	Saline
	Applications	None or moistened alginate sheet
	Dressing	Paraffin gauze or non-adherent dressing
2.	Shallow, clean, exudate	
	Cleaning	Saline
	Applications	None, alginate sheet or gel
	Dressing	Simple non-adherent or more absorbent dressing
3.	Shallow, sloughy	
	Debridement	Physical
	Cleaning	Saline or chlorhexidine
	Applications	Weak acid, gel or colloid
	Dressing	Non-adherent or colloid-impregnated
4.	Deep, clean, no exudate	
	Cleaning	Saline with irrigation if necessary
	Applications	Moistened alginate rope
	Dressing	Non-adherent
5.	Deep, clean, exudate	
	Cleaning	Saline
	Applications	Alginate rope or gel
	Dressing	Non-adherent or more absorbent
6.	Deep and sloughy	
	Debridement	Physical
	Cleaning	Saline or chlorhexidine
	Applications	Gel or colloid
	Dressing	Non-adherent or absorbent

Table 10.4 Applications and dressings.

APPLICATIONS

Desloughing agents
Weak acids
Aserbine
Variclene

Hydrogen peroxide
3% or 6% hydrogen peroxide
Hioxyl

Enzyme preparations
Varidase

Gels, colloids and polymer beads
Intrasite gel
Geliperm paste
Vigilon
Granuflex
Debrisan
Iodosorb paste

Colloid impregnated dressings
Granuflex
Tegasorb
Comfeel
Biofilm

Other osmotically active agents
Sugar paste

Cleansing agents
Sterile saline
0.05% chlorhexidine
Povidone-iodine solution
5% acetic acid
0.01% potassium permanganate
1% cetrimide

Topical antibiotic preparations
Silver sulphadiazine (Flamazine)
Metronidazole gel (Metrotop)
Mupirocin ointment (Bactroban)

Applications to promote healing
Alginates
Kaltostat
Sorbsan

For overgranulation
Hydrocortisone and neomycin cream

NON-ADHERENT DRESSINGS

Semi-absorbent
Melolin
N/A dressings
Perfron
Ete
Tricotex

Absorbent
Allevyn
Lyofoam

Activated charcoal
Actisorb Plus
Carbonet

Non-absorbent
Paraffin tulle
Paratulle
Jelonet

Povidone-iodine impregnated
Inadine

Omission of any particular preparation from this table is not intended. Similarly, inclusion of any item should not necessarily be taken as an endorsement of its value. Not all those listed are available on the NHS Drug Tariff.

11   Amputation and rehabilitation

INTRODUCTION

The idea of amputation of the leg conveys horror to the patient, relatives and staff alike. This reaction is out of proportion to the operation itself and to the debility which it involves, and is not found with many other operations or diseases that may be just as mutilating. There is almost a sense of isolation, or of being ostracized, associated with an amputee and this has deep roots in our consciousness. Perhaps this is made subtly worse by the feeling of failure experienced by doctors and nurses who may have been striving for months to save the limb.

Yet the operation should be regarded in a much more positive light. Historically, it represented the difference between life and death because secondary infection was an almost inevitable complication of the major trauma for which amputations were performed in the past. Today it represents for a diabetic the difference between continuing for many more months and years with ulcers complicated by recurrent infection and with no sign of healing, and an early return to an independent, ambulant life. For many, it needs to be done sooner, rather than later.

WHEN SHOULD AMPUTATION BE CONSIDERED?

Amputation involves removal of non-viable tissue with the object of leaving a wound which will heal.

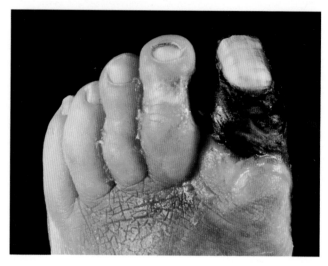

Figure 11.1 Cellulitis of the foot has been complicated by the development of gangrene in the big toe. The line of demarcation is sloughy, indicating some remaining soft tissue infection. The appearance of the rest of the foot suggests that the overall blood supply may be fairly good and amputation of the digit alone might be attempted.

The extent of the operation depends on the extent of the necrosis and the blood supply to the surrounding tissue, as well as on the choice of eventual prosthesis, whether footwear or artificial limb. As most amputations are performed because the foot is ischaemic, the possibility of improving the circulation by angio-

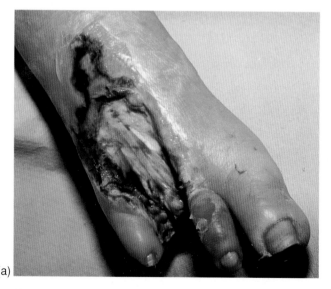

(a)

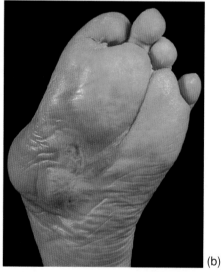

(b)

Figure 11.2(a) Ray excision of the distal metatarsals and digits will fail if the blood supply to the surrounding foot is poor. The extent of the devitalized tissue indicates that the loss of the limb is inevitable. **(b)** Successful ray excision was performed on the middle digit of this foot which is also deformed by Charcot arthropathy. The Charcot foot is a complication of neuropathy and the blood supply is normally well preserved, which is why the amputation healed well.

plasty or bypass surgery should already have been considered.

Localized surgery

The place for localized surgery is limited in diabetes because the ischaemia of the surrounding tissues means that there is a danger that the wound may not heal. It requires experience to predict which will and which will not.

If the demarcation line at the base of a digit is dry, and the toe is firmly attached to the foot, then it is usually best left in place. If, however, the line of demarcation is moist (Figure 11.1), it is almost inevitable that it will become secondarily infected at some stage.

Prophylactic administration of broad-spectrum antibiotics will not prevent such infections and there are two main treatment options:

1. to continue to dress the wound daily, to reduce the risk of secondary infection by keeping it clean and in the hope that it will eventually become dry and mummified;
2. to remove the toe if it is felt that the wound will heal.

RAY EXCISION

Ray excision involves removal of one or more toes by amputating them at the mid-metatarsal level and removing associated soft tissue. The wound is usually left open – to heal by secondary intention. A failed operation is illustrated in Figure 11.2(a); the lack of viability of the surrounding tissues is obvious. On the other hand a successful excision is demonstrated in Figure 11.2(b).

This person also had the deformity of Charcot neuropathic osteoarthropathy – a condition which is associated with increased, rather than reduced, blood flow to the foot. She actually had a bounding dorsalis pedis pulse, and the gangrene of her toe was caused by small vessel disease; there was always a good chance that the ray excision would heal.

DIGIT AMPUTATION

Amputation through the metatarsal head is less mutilating, and may be chosen in place of a ray excision if the main problem seems restricted to the digit. Such localized amputation may be the best approach to the management of extensive soft tissue infection (Figure 11.3). The site may be left either open or sewn over (Figures 11.4).

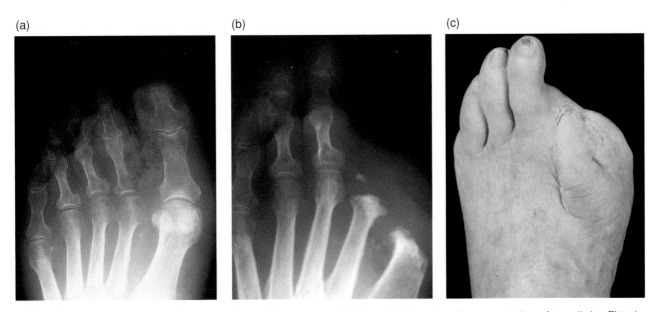

(a)   (b)   (c)

Figure 11.3(a) An X-ray showing extensive soft tissue infection with gas in the tissues. **(b)** The same foot following treatment with antibiotics and amputation of the first and second toes through the metatarsal heads.

(c) Complete healing after amputation of two digits. Fitted footwear is now necessary to prevent secondary neuropathic ulceration of the deformed foot.

When a localized amputation fails because the blood supply is insufficient to promote effective healing, then repeat local surgery usually fails as well. This is especially true if the dominant underlying problem is macrovascular disease with critically reduced flow in the larger arteries. Such people are best managed by proceeding to major amputation. Sometimes, however, the obstruction to the large vessels is less critical and delayed healing is more the result of microvascular disease. In such cases, repeat local surgery may produce a good result (Figures 11.5).

TRANSMETATARSAL AMPUTATION

Transmetatarsal amputation may be considered if the person is developing gangrene successively of one toe after another, but the progressive loss of the digits usually indicates significant macrovascular disease and more major amputation may prove inevitable. Transmetatarsal amputation was first described by Lisfranc in 1815, the year of the Battle of Waterloo.

SYME'S OPERATION

Disarticulation of the ankle was described by James Syme in 1845. It is not performed very often – even when there is a chance that an operation at that level would heal – because it is usually held that the prostheses available for below-knee amputees are preferable. However, someone who has had a successful Syme's operation is at least able to pad to the bathroom in the middle of the night without having to crawl, hop or put on an artificial leg.

COMPLICATIONS OF LOCALIZED SURGERY

Secondary neuropathic ulceration

The mutilation of the foot results in abnormal pressure distribution and this can cause either delayed healing (Figure 11.6) or the development of a new ulcer (Figure 11.7). It is essential for people to be fitted with appropriate orthoses after removal of a digit.

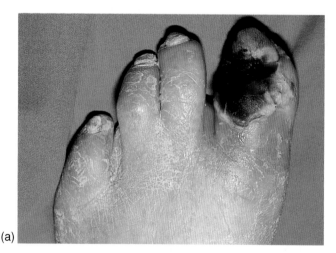

(a)

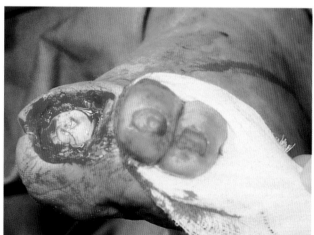

(b)

Figure 11.4(a) Extensive infection of the hallux involving both soft tissue and bone. The fourth toe has previously been removed. **(b)** Photograph taken at the time of amputation. **(c)** The same foot with the wound oversewn.

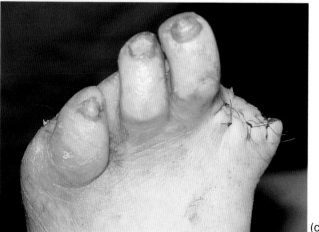

(c)

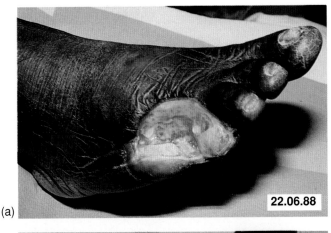

(a)

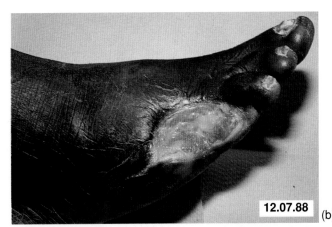

(b)

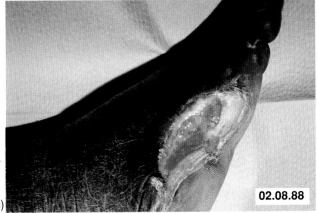

(c)

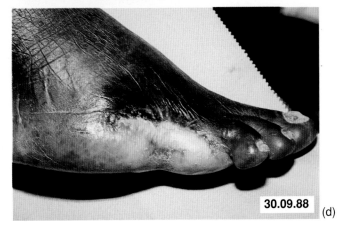

(d)

Figure 11.5(a) Wide excision of the fourth and fifth toes and their metatarsal heads has left a clean wound with fresh bleeding at the edges – indicating that the blood supply to the remaining foot is fairly good. **(b)** Rapid healing with the base filling with healthy granulation tissue and the periphery closing in. **(c)** Any callus which forms around the edge of a successful toe amputation should be removed to allow the epithelialization to continue. **(d)** The wound has completely healed. Even though the recovery from this operation was uneventful, it is notable that it took 3 months for the wound to heal.

Failure to heal

The most common complication is failure of the wound to heal. Some cases are then best managed by major amputation, whereas others are left with an unhealing wound which may persist for months, or indefinitely.

Major surgery

Amputation through the lower part of the tibia and fibula is contraindicated because the blood supply to this area is normally poor and the wound is unlikely to heal. For this reason major surgery is undertaken at, or around, the knee.

INDICATIONS FOR MAJOR SURGERY

It is usually obvious when a foot is so ischaemic that it will never heal (Figure 11.8).

A major amputation should be recommended, providing that:

1. the patient would withstand the procedure;
2. the loss of the limb would not leave him/her more incapacitated than if s/he were to keep it;
3. s/he agrees that it is necessary.

Major amputation is occasionally performed as an emergency for critical limb ischaemia (painful white leg) from atherosclerosis or embolus, or for overwhelming sepsis. It may also be performed on younger people with major deformity from neuropathic osteoarthropathy (see Chapter 7).

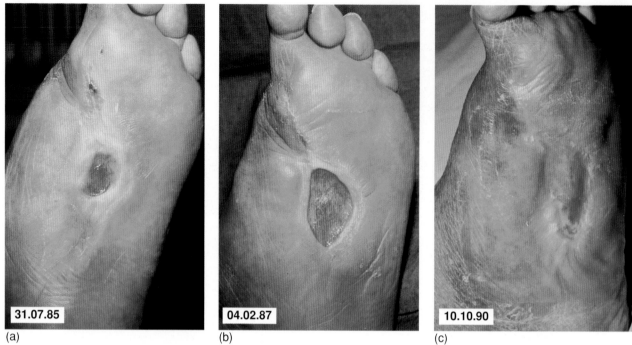

(a)   (b)   (c)

Figure 11.6(a) July 1985. Neuropathic ulcer following ray excision of the hallux 2 months earlier. **(b)** February 1987. The ulcer persists despite frequent dressings and attempted grafting. **(c)** October 1990. The ulcer eventually healed.

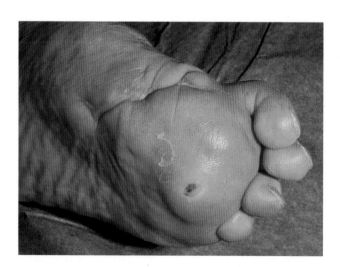

Figure 11.7 Secondary neuropathic ulceration will follow otherwise successful amputation of a digit unless fitted footwear is provided.

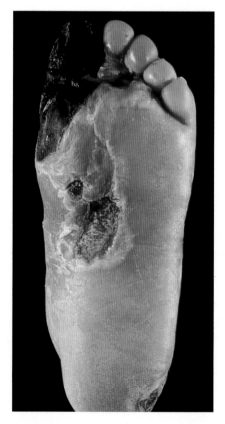

Figure 11.8 The spread of gangrene from the hallux to the second and third toes, and the involvement of the instep and the heel indicate that this foot cannot be saved.

CONTRAINDICATIONS TO MAJOR SURGERY

Non-compliance

Some patients cannot accept the idea of losing a limb and will often say that they would prefer to die. While many change their minds with time and sensitive care, especially if the foot becomes more necrotic and smelly from infection, some do not. It is easy to understand such an attitude, which is based partly on fear and partly on blind hope that the limb may improve on its own. Their wishes must be respected but they are usually condemned to a miserable last few months.

Medically unfit

Patients may be unfit for surgery because of co-existing disease such as ischaemic heart disease. Surgery could not be considered for a man with extensive ischaemic lesions of both feet (Figure 11.9) because he had had a recent myocardial infarction complicated by severe low-output failure.

He was managed instead by regular chiropody, with piecemeal removal of dead tissue. He kept both legs and was able to potter about as much as his heart would allow until he died in his sleep 2 years later.

Second amputation

Some 20% of survivors who have an amputation will go on to lose the other leg within 3 years. This second operation has far greater implications for their independence and mobility, and for their self-esteem (Figure 11.10).

The loss of both legs requires a major alteration of balance and everyday tasks such as dressing, washing, using the toilet and transferring from bed to chair become very difficult. An older person may find it impossible to adapt to the change – especially if the illness which preceded the surgery resulted in months of immobility which would inevitably be associated with muscle wasting. A second amputation should be avoided at all costs in someone who has little chance of returning to anything resembling an independent existence with two prostheses. It is better for an elderly person to die with one leg with a hole in it than to die with no legs at all.

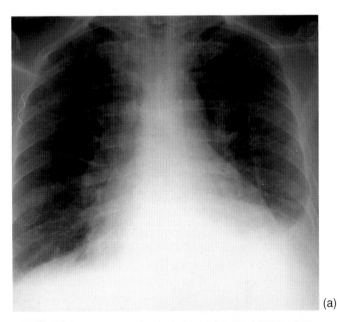
(a)

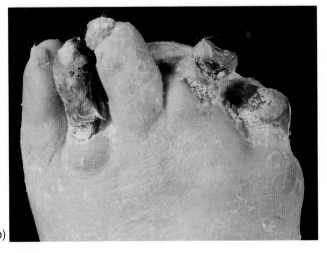
(b)

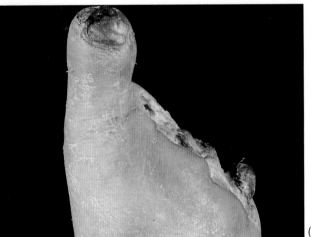
(c)

Figure 11.9(a) The chest X-ray of a man with diabetic gangrene. He had gross congestive cardiac failure with cardiomegaly and pleural effusion following a myocardial infarction, which meant that he was unfit for general anaesthesia. **(b)** and **(c)** The extensive gangrene of his toes was managed simply by regular chiropody.

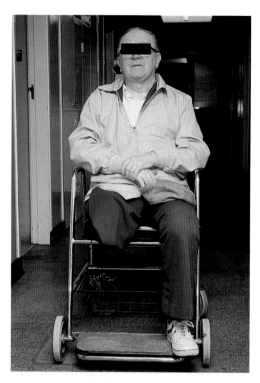

Figure 11.10 This man has had below-knee surgery on the left and an above-knee operation on the right. As a bilateral amputee who previously lived alone he is trapped by his incapacity in the environment of hospitals and of health care professionals.

BELOW-KNEE AMPUTATION

The site is selected far enough below the knee to allow the fashioning of a useful artificial limb, but at the same time high enough to ensure healing (Figure 11.11). Large flaps of soft tissue are preserved to pad the amputated bone. The wound is oversewn.

ABOVE-KNEE AMPUTATION

Amputation above the knee is done either as a primary procedure in someone whose blood supply is known to be so poor that below-knee surgery would be unlikely to heal, or as a secondary procedure when an earlier operation has failed. Both above- and below-knee amputation are performed under antibiotic cover.

GRITTI–STOKES AMPUTATION

This approach to amputation through the knee was described separately in Italy (1857) and the UK (1870) but is not favoured nowadays because of the difficulty of providing a suitable prosthesis. If a normal length femur is capped with the proximal end of a jointed artificial lower limb, the eventual position of the 'knee' joint is too low. The operation should only be considered in those in whom a prosthesis is not planned and who will always be wheelchair-dependent.

THE PROCESS OF REHABILITATION

The process of physical and psychological rehabilitation is protracted. It requires a tremendous investment of time and effort and some never complete it. The process is made easier if the patient is managed in a specialist rehabilitation centre, but this is rarely possible. More often than not, patients are managed on an acute medical, surgical or geriatric ward where the skills of doctors and nurses are directed more to the management of the acutely ill, and where other professional input is not always as coordinated as it

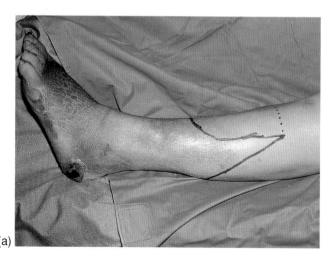
(a)

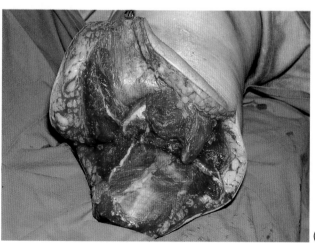
(b)

Figure 11.11(a) The incision for a below-knee amputation is planned such that a pad of soft tissue is left to protect the stump. **(b)** The operation site before being oversewn at surgery.

might be. The length of the process and the feeling of being a burden to hard-worked nursing staff may increase the sense of isolation felt by some, and may exacerbate any tendency to depression which follows mutilating surgery.

The perioperative phase

If the wound heals well, the stitches are removed after 2–3 weeks. During this time the accent of rehabilitation is placed on simple exercises to maintain muscle strength as much as possible. At the same time the options for care after discharge from hospital are explored with the family and carers. If the wound becomes infected and breaks down, this phase can become very protracted and demoralizing for the patient.

Later rehabilitation

Once they have recovered from the operation and are able to undertake simple tasks of daily living, their ability to manage during a home visit is assessed by an occupational therapist, physiotherapist and/or social worker (Figure 11.12(a) and (b)). Alterations are made to doorways, passages and stairs to facilitate the use of a wheelchair (Figure 11.12(c)), and beds may need to be moved downstairs and commodes provided. The patient may need other social support, including community nursing, Meals on Wheels, etc.

Physiotherapy will continue in the physiotherapy department of the hospital where the operation was done and will be aimed at increasing confidence and mobility as much as possible. When the swelling around the stump has settled, they start walking practice with a blown-up splint (Figure 11.13).

PROSTHESES

The provision of prostheses is arranged at a regional limb-fitting centre and can be undertaken only when the stump has largely settled. Even so, progressive remoulding takes place over the months and years and new moulds need to be made from time to time for the cup which fits into the top of the prosthesis (Figure 11.14).

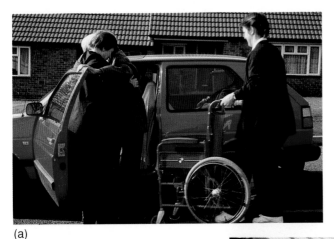

(a)

Figure 11.12(a) A home visit enables occupational therapist, physiotherapist and social worker to assess the patient's capacity for independent existence and requirements for support. **(b)** The drive and front door steps may need to be modified to enable a less agile person to gain access with either a frame or wheelchair. **(c)** Many passages are too narrow to accommodate a wheelchair.

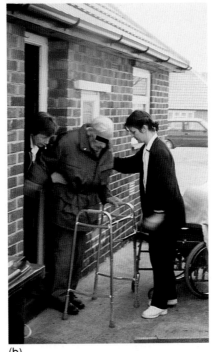

(b)

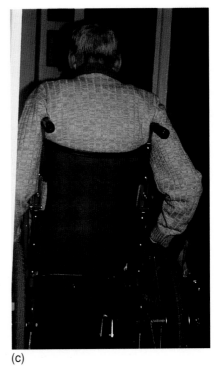

(c)

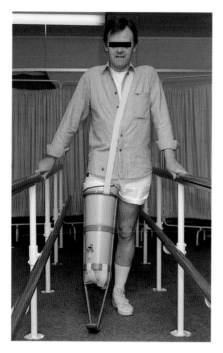

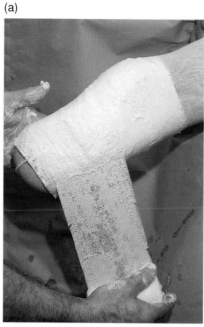

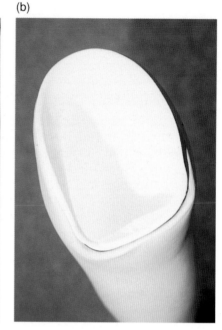

Figure 11.13 A temporary inflatable splint can be used to start walking practice once the initial swelling of the operation has started to resolve.

Figure 11.14(a) A plaster of Paris template is taken of the stump and used to make the cup which fits into the top of the prosthesis. **(b)** Replacement cups can be fitted as the stump continues to remodel and change shape.

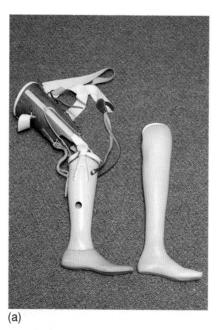

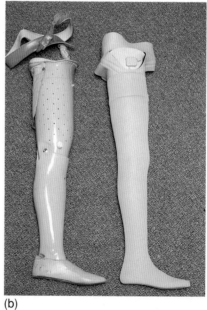

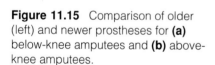

Figure 11.15 Comparison of older (left) and newer prostheses for **(a)** below-knee amputees and **(b)** above-knee amputees.

The prostheses which are available for both below- and above-knee amputees are lightweight, flexible and easily attached, with the cup which has been moulded to the shape of the stump being slotted into the top (Figure 11.15). Once a person has adapted to their use, they can regain much of their independence. Even a bilateral amputee can learn to manage stairs and can return to full-time employment (Figure 11.16).

Problems in the rehabilitation phase

PSYCHOLOGICAL AND SOCIAL

It is at this stage that the major psychological effect of the operation is felt – the realization that they will never be the same again.

These are the feelings of a 63-year-old man recovering in hospital from his second amputation.

> They told me at the end of January and I had the operation 10 days later. I felt very bad. I was suicidal. I was in a room on my own and there was no-one to talk to. I feel helpless. I can do lots of things, but not things like going to the toilet, that's the worst problem for me. It's very degrading. If I knew then what I know now, I would have asked them just to amputate my toes. Nobody explained. I'm going for a home visit later this week but I'm anxious. I can't go back to my old place. I should imagine I'll be very lonely living on my own. I feel very, very lonely and a bit frightened. I'm not a young man. I used to do a bit of gardening. I like sport on the television, the racing; I like a few bob on.

There is a critical time which follows discharge from hospital, at which the patient may feel most isolated and rejected. They have lost the support of 24-hour nursing care, and the reality of their immobility and dependence on others is, literally, brought home to them. This is particularly true for an elderly couple, or for an elderly person living on their own, who were previously only just managing to cling onto an independent existence. The coordination of caring support which they need is not always available.

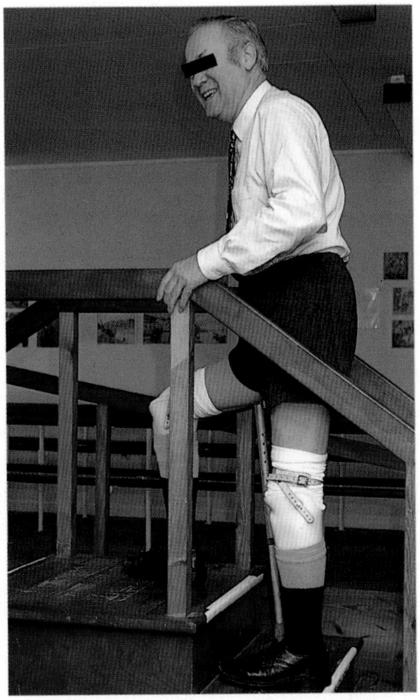

Even those who are determined to adapt to using an artificial leg may feel thwarted by the inevitable slowness of the process, and the need to travel frequently by ambulance to a limb-fitting centre (which may be many miles away) may sap the strength of an elderly person. Younger people may have less of a physical problem coping with prostheses, but the psychological reaction may still be severe. They have to adapt to becoming something which they had not thought about seriously before – disabled.

These feelings were expressed by the young man whose injury was illustrated in Figure 3.9 and who underwent a below-knee amputation after 7 months in an orthopaedic ward.

> When I was told that my leg was to be amputated, I felt nothing emotionally. After the amputation I still felt nothing, and then I received my false limb. That was when everything hit home. I hated the fact that I wasn't like everyone else. I hated the false limb and wouldn't even try it on for two days. Then I realized that either I spent the rest of my life in a wheelchair or learned to live with it. I chose the latter.

Some harbour a deep-seated doubt that the operation might not really have been necessary and that if only they had waited, the leg could have been saved.

PHYSICAL

Although phantom-limb pain is relatively uncommon, diabetic amputees usually retain the sensation of the leg 'being there'. The result can mean that in the early days they may sometimes forget that the leg has been lost and when they are not wearing their prosthesis, they may get up from bed or a chair and try to walk on the missing leg. The result is a painful injury to the stump (Figure 11.17) and, often, a secondary psychological reaction to the reality of their situation.

The stump may also develop secondary neuropathic ulceration, which will need to be managed by regular cleansing until healed and refashioning of the cup (Figure 11.18).

Figure 11.16 A bilateral amputee can regain considerable independence of movement.

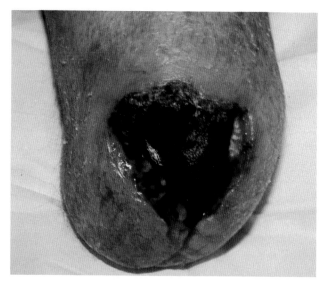

Figure 11.17 Abrasion to the stump caused by the amputee forgetting that his leg was no longer there. He was not wearing his prosthesis when he got up from a chair and tried to walk across the room.

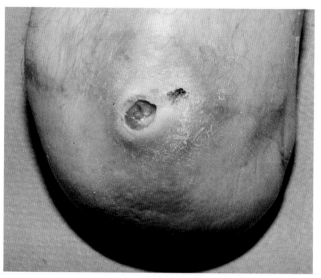

Figure 11.18 A neuropathic ulcer on the stump – caused by unnoticed rubbing on the cup of the prosthesis.

OUTCOME AFTER AMPUTATION

There are few data on survival following amputation of the leg for diabetes. Data from Newcastle report a 50% 2-year survival of 48 patients with diabetes undergoing amputation between 1989 and 1991. Our own experience over the last 10 years is similar, and is summarized in Figure 11.19. Survival for women is worse because they are on average 10 years older than men at the time of first amputation. Of amputees who survive, in both Newcastle and Nottingham, 20% will lose the other leg within 3 years.

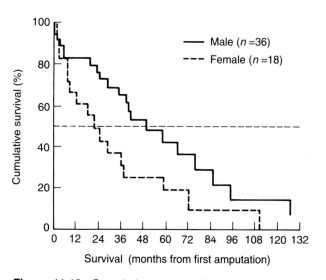

Figure 11.19 Cumulative survival of 54 diabetics following lower limb amputation in Nottingham between 1982 and 1994.

12 Prevention of foot ulcers

Some people with diabetes are predisposed to the development of foot problems. There are three reasons for this:

1. hyperglycaemia, which impairs healing;
2. complications of diabetes, such as vasculopathy and neuropathy;
3. problems unrelated to diabetes – immobility, being socially disadvantaged or unaware of the risks.

When an ulcer occurs, it may heal or it may persist. If it persists, it may worsen and lead to amputation of the leg with all the devastating consequences for the patient. Thus, preventive strategies have to be directed at the factors which **predispose** a person to ulceration, to the factors which **precipitate** one and to those which allow it to **perpetuate**.

Effective education is crucial. This implies education of both the patient and the professionals looking after him/her. Effective education has to be targeted and repeated as often as necessary; the objective is not just to increase knowledge but to induce a change of behaviour.

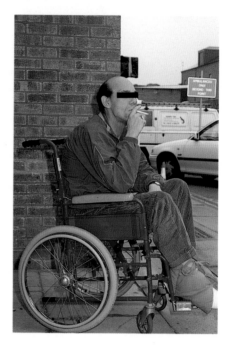

Figure 12.1 The single most important aspect of foot care education for a young diabetic is advice about not smoking.

EDUCATION OF PEOPLE WITH DIABETES

The young and fit

PREDISPOSITION

The risk of developing an ulcer in later life is less if the onset of vasculopathy and neuropathy is reduced. This will be achieved by better control of blood glucose and attention to exercise and diet, but the chances are that the young diabetic is already doing as much as they can (or will) in this direction. Exhortations to a recalcitrant teenager to manage their diabetes better in order to prevent gangrene in 40 years time is likely to produce little more than a metaphorical shrug of the shoulders. However, the single fact that the young **must** appreciate is the danger of smoking: young diabetics who smoke are far more likely to get problems with their feet than those who do not (Figure 12.1).

AVOIDING BREAKS IN THE SKIN

There are three factors which break the skin in this group: (1) tinea; (2) ingrowing toenail; and (3) an accident. Those with normal sensation will be aware of athlete's foot because of the pricking pain it causes, but they should be taught to check for it, and those who have recurrent infections should have a tube of antifungal cream available at home so that they can treat any outbreak as early as possible. Ingrowing

toenails will be similarly symptomatic and should be treated along conventional lines.

The vast majority of breaks will, however, result from an accident – and accidents are, by their nature, unavoidable. Thus, there is little point in giving too much prescriptive advice to young people about how often they should wash their feet, how they should cut their toenails and whether or not they should walk barefoot. A young diabetic with good circulation is no more at risk from a cut on their foot than a non-diabetic, and an over-didactic approach to education may lead to alienation. A 22-year-old girl who is going on holiday to a Greek island should not be told to wear 'sensible' shoes on the beach – at a time when she may be wearing nothing else! She would not take any notice, anyway.

All people over the age of about 30 should have their feet examined annually to look for those who might be becoming 'at risk', but also to reinforce the educational process.

The older, fit person

All people over the age of 55 should have access to specific education about foot care. This is the group which needs to take special precautions: the mean age of men who have an amputation is 64, and the mean age of women is 72. They can be taught on a one-to-one basis at the time of their annual check, but they can also be taught successfully in groups. Many elderly people enjoy the social side of group educational sessions at the surgery, and it becomes an opportunity also for people to discuss other aspects of diabetes management.

PREDISPOSITION

Older people need to learn that they are at increased risk – simply because ulcers are more likely to occur with advancing age. They need to take sensible general precautions (e.g. regular foot care, well-fitting shoes, avoid walking barefoot, comfortable slippers around the house (Figure 12.2)) and they need to get into the habit of inspecting their feet each day to look for the first sign of trouble. If they cannot see well, or they cannot bend down to examine their feet because of obesity or arthritis, then they need to get somebody else to do it for them.

AVOIDING BREAKS IN THE SKIN

The main difference from advice given to the younger person is the emphasis placed on regular foot care, and those who are unable to look after their own feet should have easy access to a state-registered chiropodist (Figure 12.3).

The patient whose feet are 'at risk'

People whose feet are 'at risk' because of vasculopathy or neuropathy or both need to be told that their feet are at risk, and why (Figure 12.4).

Their records should be clearly flagged (Figure 12.5), and their feet should be examined in the surgery on a regular basis.

In general terms people are as reluctant to take their shoes and socks off to have their feet examined as doctors and nurses are to do the examining, and a

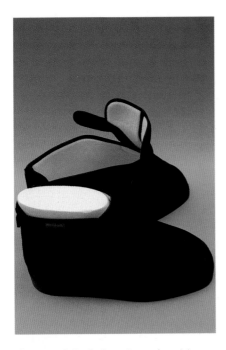

Figure 12.2 Soft and comfortable padded slippers should be worn about the house, and ones like those shown should be provided also for people in hospital whose own shoes will not fit over any dressings they may have. Many patients with active ulcers are left to pad barefoot about the ward with no covering on their feet except their bandages.

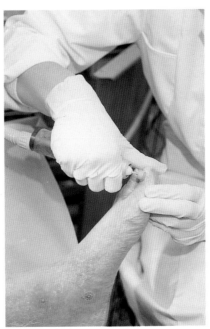

Figure 12.3 All older people should have easy access to the skills of a state-registered chiropodist.

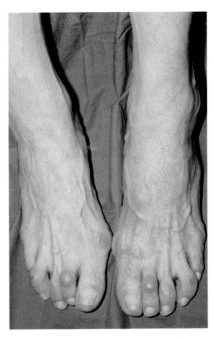

Figure 12.4 Recognition of the foot 'at risk' is an essential skill for all doctors and nurses. This woman has misshapen feet which are affected by both neuropathy and vasculopathy. The skin of the forefoot looks generally a bit thin and ischaemic, and the thinned skin on the dorsum of the left fourth toe is reddened. There is a corn on the right second and build-up of callus on the left second toe. There are shallow neuropathic ulcers on the first and fourth toes on the right.

133

pattern has to be established whereby it becomes part of the usual consultation. If the doctor or nurse simply asks 'Do you have any problems with your feet?', the patient may well deny the existence of any ulcer that they might have.

PREDISPOSITION

There is little that can be done about any established vasculopathy or neuropathy which puts the older person at risk, and the main effort lies in preventing a break in the skin which might then be slow to heal.

AVOIDING BREAKS IN THE SKIN

Foot care

Paradoxically, the person with onychogryphosis (see Figure 8.23), or with long and unkempt toenails, is not at as great a risk of losing their limb as might be thought (Figure 12.6).

Toenails require oxygen and nutrients to grow and do not grow quickly in the presence of ischaemia. As it is ischaemia which is the factor most likely to delay healing, it follows that any abrasion caused by such nails will heal quickly. It is worth noting in passing that we have a tendency to be critical of people with onychogryphosis ('How could they let their feet get in such a state?') without necessarily understanding the reasons why the nails become so grossly thickened, or appreciate how difficult it is to cut them.

Sensory neuropathy

Someone with peripheral sensory neuropathy should be made aware of the numbness of their feet and should be taught to be especially careful about minor trauma which they might not notice. Thus they may not realize that new shoes are too tight or that they are rubbing a blister (Figures 12.7 and 12.8).

They may not even notice that they have trodden on a drawing pin and that it is going through their shoe (see Figure 3.12).

They should also get into the habit of feeling in their shoes before they put them on in case something has dropped into them, or the insole has become crumpled. When they have a bath, they

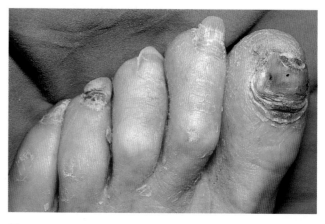

Figure 12.6 Unkempt nails do not pose as much of a risk to the foot as might at first be thought.

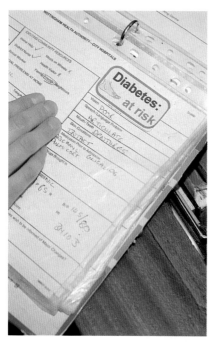

Figure 12.5 (left) Clear flagging of records is essential and must be obvious to all involved in care – doctor, chiropodist, nurse, receptionist.

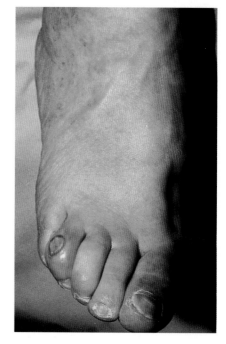

Figure 12.7 (right) This man has peripheral sensory neuropathy and was not aware that he had rubbed the sore on his right fourth toe.

should test the temperature with their hand and forearm, and not their feet. They should learn that there is a risk of burns if they doze in front of the fire, and hot water bottles can burn or blister the skin – even when protected with a woolly cover (Figure 12.9).

Motor neuropathy and limited joint mobility

The presence of motor neuropathy, limited joint mobility and other deformity may determine the need for fitted footwear, but it is the responsibility of the professional to recognize this (see below).

Ischaemia

The presence of ischaemia poses an even greater threat than that of neuropathy, because it is the ischaemic foot which is at particular risk of infection and of gangrene. People should be encouraged to wash their feet every day – as much to ensure that they look at them as for any other reason. Those with dry skin should moisten it with E45, moisturising cream or hand cream. If cracks can be prevented in this way, it will reduce the incidence of infection.

PROMOTING EARLY HEALING

The single most important piece of advice to be given and stressed is the need to seek help for any ulcer at the earliest possible opportunity. They should be seen within 24 hours by a doctor, nurse or chiropodist with specific knowledge about the

management of such problems, and they should be seen again at frequent intervals to ensure that it is getting better. Unfortunately, people tend to delay seeking help, either because they are not aware of the potential seriousness of the situation or because they are aware and simply hope that the problem will go away.

What to teach

Most educational programmes concentrate on the rather bland footcare advice given above, and it is found in the many printed leaflets which are available (Figure 12.10).

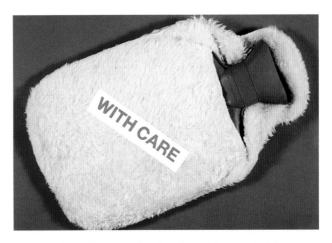

Figure 12.9 Hot water bottles should be used with great caution.

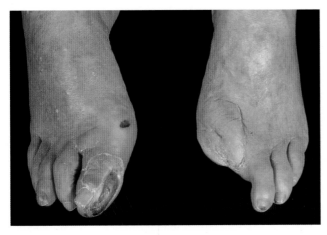

Figure 12.8 This lady had had extensive soft tissue infection of her left foot successfully treated by amputation of the first and second toes (Figure 11.3), but soon afterwards made the mistake of walking around all day with the wrong shoes on the wrong feet and this caused the lesion seen. Fortunately, it healed with careful nursing and chiropody.

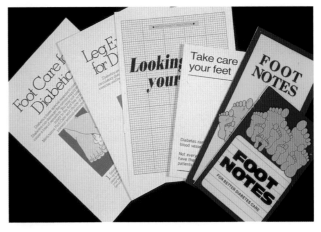

Figure 12.10 Printed footcare literature tends to offer rather bland, prescriptive advice. It should be used as an adjunct to one-to-one and group teaching, not in place of it.

Such leaflets should only be used as an adjunct to personal instruction, and not instead of it. Unfortunately, people do not always learn what they have been taught and even when they do they may find it hard to change old habits. It is particularly surprising that people do not always learn from the experience of having an ulcer: all too often they get others for the same, usually avoidable, reason.

There is evidence, however, that in those who have already had one major amputation, the likelihood of losing the second leg can be significantly reduced if all patients undergo an intensive education programme – especially one in which they are shown explicit pictures. Perhaps we should be more aggressive in the techniques we use.

Adverse effects of patient education

It should be remembered that the educational process may have an adverse effect. If the person is taught that it is their responsibility to try and prevent ulceration, they may feel guilty when it occurs. If they think it is their fault, they may be more reluctant to reveal it to a doctor, nurse or chiropodist. For this reason every educational session should finish with the reminder that the most important thing to do is to ask for help as quickly as possible whenever a lesion is noticed (Table 12.1).

EDUCATION OF THE PROFESSIONAL

When we undertook a retrospective survey of the causes of a large number of foot ulcers, we found that substandard management by professionals was twice as likely to contribute to the onset or deterioration of a lesion as carelessness on the part of the patient themselves. Nevertheless, formal postgraduate training in this area is universally lacking – even though the majority of ulcers present to, and are managed by, non-specialist doctors and nurses working in primary care. Such professionals need clear guidance.

The general practitioner

Family doctors need to understand the contribution made to lesions by infection, ischaemia and neuropathy, and how to determine the priority of management. They should be encouraged to seek advice by telephone and to refer urgently if appropriate (Table 12.2).

They need to know who in the area has the greatest interest in the field (generally speaking, in the UK this will be a diabetologist, rather than a vascular surgeon). Once again, it is the need for expert assessment at the earliest opportunity which is paramount: delayed referral may result in avoidable deterioration in the ulcer. If the doctor elects to manage the ulcer without referral, arrangements must be made for early and repeated review.

Doctors and nurses also need to be able to detect the foot which is 'at risk', and to recognize when action needs to be taken to prevent ulceration occurring (Table 12.2). Thus the detection of a neuropathic foot with callus should prompt referral for regular chiropody and consideration of the need for fitted footwear. Similarly, a patient with limited joint mobility affecting the first toe may be considered for shoes with a rocker-bar, or rocker soles, which will result in less pressure being taken by the big toe during normal walking (Figure 12.11).

Nurses working in primary care

The work of doctors and nurses overlaps in the field of diabetes care and much of what is true for doctors (see above) is true also for nurses. However, nurses

---

Table 12.1 Essential requirements of an educational programme

- It should be targeted at a particular group.
- The content should be appropriate for that group.
- It should be repeated.
- The most important item to be emphasized is the need for urgent expert assessment.

Table 12.2 What health care professionals should know

- How to recognize the foot which is 'at risk'.
- The need for early and repeated assessment of any ulcer.
- That referral to a specialist unit should take place earlier rather than later.
- Which local unit has the greatest interest in foot problems.
- Telephone numbers of relevant contacts.

obviously need, more than doctors, to have a working knowledge of the different types of dressings and applications. Nurses should have the contact numbers of other specialists (nurse, chiropodist or doctor) to whom they can turn for advice.

Receptionists

Receptionists need to learn the urgency with which foot ulcers need to be assessed, and they also need to know whose feet are at special risk. Patients who contact the surgery for help should receive it on the same day.

Chiropodists

Chiropodists are experts in the field, by the nature of their training. However, they suffer from professional isolation which results partly from tradition and partly from a separate administrative network. Chiropodists should be encouraged to establish closer contact with doctors and nurses working in both primary and secondary care.

Doctors in hospitals

Doctors are reluctant to consider early referral and tend to seek advice only when a situation is obviously not improving. This barrier may adversely affect the outcome of a diabetic foot ulcer which requires the multidisciplinary skills of a specialist team. All too often, diabetic ulcers are managed by other specialists (orthopaedic, plastic surgical, general surgical, general medical, geriatric) who may not be aware of the need to consider cross-referral. Even in hospitals where a specialist diabetic foot care team exists, our evidence is that some three-quarters of amputations in diabetics are performed under the supervision of other units. Surgeons who remove one or more toes often do not foresee the likelihood of secondary neuropathic ulcers occurring and rarely refer for fitted footwear.

Junior medical staff may also be ignorant of the specialist services available – especially if they have been appointed only recently.

Nurses in hospitals

Nurses in nursing homes and hospitals need to be specifically taught to recognize 'at risk' feet (Figure 12.4), and to take special precautions to protect them when they have been identified. Pressure sores such as that illustrated in Figure 12.12 can arise very quickly in the immobilized patient with ischaemic feet and protective measures must be used at all times.

These include 'sheepskin' rugs, special mattresses, padded boots and pillows on footstools (Figure

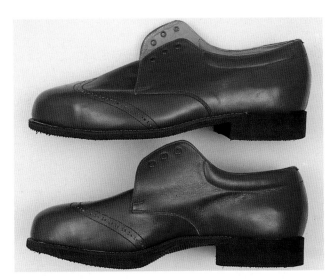

Figure 12.11 The effect of a rocker sole is to reduce the propulsive force required from the big toe during the 'toe-off' phase of walking. This will reduce the risk of secondary neuropathic ulceration if the toe is made inflexible by limited joint mobility.

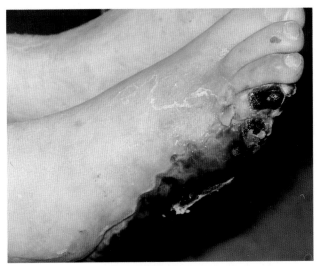

Figure 12.12 Disastrous pressure sores can occur very quickly in the elderly person immobilized by ill-health. They are particularly likely following stroke because patients are even less likely to be aware of increased pressure on the affected side, and may be completely unable to alter it for themselves.

12.13). Even a pair of thick woolly socks is better than nothing.

Sometimes professionals forget to protect the feet because they are concentrating on other problems which may be more important at the time. Protective boots may be provided, but not worn (Figure 12.13(d)). Foot ulcers are common on the feet of diabetics with vascular disease who have had a stroke, as well as on surgical wards. The heel is at special risk if it is unprotected during prolonged general anaesthesia.

ASSESSMENT FOR THE PROVISION OF FITTED FOOTWEAR

Selection of patients for orthoses

The provision of proper footwear is an essential part of prevention of ulceration in the diabetic foot. It is usually arranged by referral from a specialist clinic to an orthotist (either NHS-employed or contracted). Many different types of shoe are available but the broad types which are provided fall into the following categories:

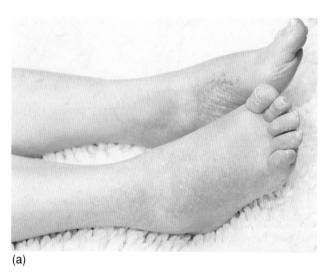

(a)

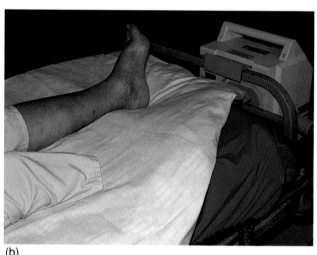

(b)

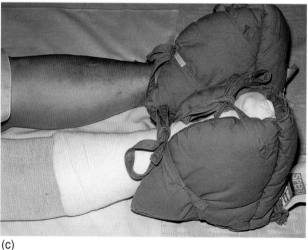

(c)

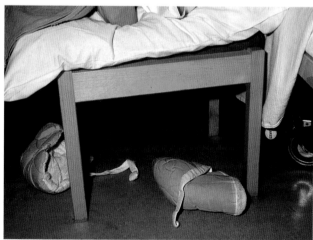

(d)

Figure 12.13(a) A 'sheepskin' rug will help to prevent ulceration of the heel. Note that this patient has dislocation of the right first metatarsophalangeal joint, presumably from neuropathy. **(b)** This man has already demonstrated his predisposition to foot ulcers and has had a below-knee amputation on the right. The left heel is being protected by using an air-filled mattress. **(c)** Effective padding of the heels with padded boots may be required to protect heels, malleoli and sides of the foot. Such boots have disadvantages, however: they are difficult to keep in place and difficult to walk with – even for the shortest trip around the bed. **(d)** Even when foot protectors are provided in hospitals, they may not always be used. This shows a pair neglected under a low table beside the patient's bed.

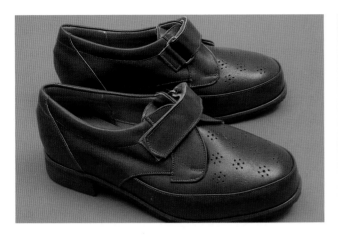

Figure 12.14 Shoes for a patient who has had neuropathic ulcers.

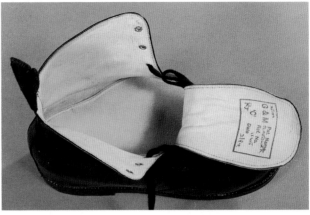

Figure 12.15 This shoe was made to accomodate a foot grossly distorted by Charcot arthropathy.

1. soft slippers to accommodate an active ulcer with its dressings;
2. shoes for the patient with a predisposition to neuropathic ulceration, with peripheral sensory neuropathy and clawing of the foot – these should be in soft material, and deep and broad enough to accommodate the foot while still being firm enough on the foot to prevent blisters and ulcers arising from shearing forces (Figure 12.14);
3. shoes for the patient with a grossly deformed foot – the same principles apply to the provision of shoes for someone with a foot deformed by, for example, Charcot osteoarthropathy, trauma or congenital malformation, but the shoes may need to be bespoke (Figure 12.15);
4. shoes for someone with peripheral vascular disease – shoes may need to be provided also for the person whose skin is liable to damage from minor trauma; such shoes are especially soft, but must be firm enough to prevent ulceration from shearing forces;
5. rocker bars may be applied to the sole of the shoe if there is limited flexibility of the hallux – from arthritis, previous osteomyelitis or diabetic limited joint mobility.

ADVICE FOR THOSE WHO PREFER TO USE THEIR OWN SHOES

People who reasonably prefer to use their own shoes should be shown the principles involved and encouraged to follow common sense more than the dictates of fashion. Soft, well-padded trainers are as good for many people as fitted orthoses.

PRACTICAL AND ETHICAL ISSUES

The provision of proper footwear is an essential part of management, but the financial and practical issues of this facility have not yet been fully debated. Shoes are currently provided in the UK by hospital specialist units for some of the patients referred to them – which represents a small fraction of the total. Nevertheless, the cost of this to the budget of a large district hospital is over £40 000 annually (1992 prices). If such units were to provide an open-ended commitment to all in the district who need fitted footwear (which includes repairs, replacements, reinforced workboots, brown pairs and black pairs, etc.), the cost would soon be astronomical and the specialist diabetic foot clinic (or occupational therapy department) would start to resemble a shoe shop. It is possible that if costs were to be borne by the patient or the budget of the general practitioner, then fewer people would have them.

Moreover, there are ethical issues which will arise as the climate of litigation increases. Health care professionals should foresee the possibility of legal action being taken – either for failing to recommend the provision of shoes or for providing ones which, as occasionally happens, do not fit well and are associated with the development of a new lesion.

13 Foot ulcers in perspective

And Asa in the thirty and ninth year of his reign was diseased in his feet, until his disease was exceeding great: yet in his disease he sought not to the Lord, but to the physicians,

And Asa slept with his fathers, and died in the one and fortieth year of his reign.

2 Chronicles 16, 12-13

This passage is often quoted in reviews of the management of diabetic gangrene, but it contains a double irony. The biblical author was unfair on the professionals of the day because there were, presumably, relatively few things that the physicians in Judah **could** do apart from put their faith in the Lord. Furthermore, the outcome for King Asa was really quite good: even today we know that only 60% of people survive for 2 years after amputation of the leg for (diabetic) gangrene. Although significant advances have been made – introduction of antibiotics, management of neuropathic ulcers, improvement in general health – we remain relatively impotent in the face of critical limb ischaemia. In many cases the outcome is unrelated to professional input and there is little that some of our patients can do – other, that is, than rely on their faith.

PREVALENCE OF FOOT PROBLEMS

Ulcers

Community surveys have demonstrated that approximately 7% of people with diabetes will have a foot ulcer at some stage, and we can anticipate that this figure will rise as the population grows older. During our own survey of a population of 200 000, with an estimated 4000 people with diabetes, we identified 41 with ulcers being actively managed by community nursing services during a single week. In other words, one diabetic in every 100 has an active ulcer at any one time. In the same survey we found that only 11 of the 41 (27%) were attending a specialist clinic.

Amputation

It is surprisingly difficult to identify the number of people who undergo amputation of the lower limb for diabetes. UK Department of Health statistics record only those referred for fitting of an artificial limb, which excludes those who are not thought suitable for a prosthesis, as well as those who die in the perioperative phase. Furthermore, many people are recorded as having an amputation for ischaemia without the contribution made by diabetes being acknowledged. However, a number of community surveys suggest that in Northern Europe there are between 60 and 100 amputations of the lower limb

performed each year for diabetes per million total population. If we assume a prevalence of diabetes of 2%, then we can calculate that one diabetic in 250 will lose a limb each year.

There are equally few data on survival after amputation, but our own figures are summarized in Table 13.1.

If these figures are worse than others published several years ago it may reflect the fact that amputation is performed increasingly only for untreatable ischaemia, and the people who undergo the operation are older and more likely to have significant cardiac and cerebrovascular disease. Of those who survive for 3 years, 20% will lose the other leg as well, the mean interval between first and second amputation being 18 months.

Table 13.1 Survival following first major amputation of the lower limb (data based on experience in Nottingham 1982–92)

	Percentage survival				
Years	1	2	3	4	5
Male	76	67	50	35	22
Female	67	50	40	30	20
Total	73	61	47	33	21

Mean age at operation Male: 63.6 ± 10.0 (SD) years
Female: 72.3 ± 11.1 years

COSTS

The immediate hospital cost of an amputation is between £8000 and £10 000, but the hidden costs of amputation, of the ulcer which predisposes to it and the rehabilitation process which follows are vast. Any estimate will be an underestimate.

Costs of health and community services

Some of the itemized costs involved are listed in Table 13.2.

Given that the median duration of any ulcer is 16 weeks, and that the median number of visits to each patient each week by a community nurse is 2.0, and that at any one time there are 200 such cases per million population, it is apparent that the costs are great.

Items not listed in Table 13.2 include transport costs (upon which the majority are dependent), chiropody, antibiotics, investigations (angiography

Table 13.2 Estimates of some of the unit costs involved in diabetes care (1994 prices)

	£
In-patient hospital stay for one day	150.00
Outpatient consultation	50.00
Community nurse visit	20.00
GP consultation	10.00
Dressings	2.00

and other imaging), treatments (angioplasty, bypass surgery), plaster casts, shoe-fitting, physiotherapy, home assessments and modification where necessary and provision of home support (Meals on Wheels, visits by diabetes specialist nurses to the home or the surgery, community nursing other than for dressings, home help, etc.).

Costs to the patient

Apart from the horror of losing a limb, or being frightened of the possibility of doing so, there are major psychological and financial costs. In the first category comes the loss of independence of an elderly person who was managing to maintain a marginally independent existence in their own home. They and their spouse may have to move from the home they have occupied for 40 years and/or they may become dependent for support on others. Each ulcer requires many visits either by or to a nurse or chiropodist, and trips to hospital may involve hours of travel and waiting. Apart from that the person may become trapped in the house, unable to get out because of immobility, or unwilling to go out because they have been told to 'rest the foot as much as possible'. Depression is commonplace.

Younger people may lose their jobs and find it harder to adapt to the role of being an invalid. They will resent the loss of mobility more. Support services are geared less to the younger person with permanent disability than they are for the elderly.

Costs to the family and carers

Costs to the family and relatives are often ignored, but are just as great. They include the costs of travelling to hospital – either to bring the patient or to visit them – possible loss of employment to care for them at home, loss of privacy and independence by bringing a disabled relative to live in their own home, the costs of minor conversions, provision of aids and the loss of much of their own free time.

The psychological costs to the spouse involve also the distress caused by the incapacity of their partner and, possibly, frustration at their own inability to cope through age and weakness. On occasion, partners – and particularly wives – may feel guilt that they may have made a lesion worse, either by not having the courage to help the nurses by doing some of the dressings themselves or by having done some of the dressings and feeling that they may have done them incorrectly. These fears are rarely expressed.

INEFFICIENCIES IN THE MANAGEMENT OF FOOT LESIONS

One of the greatest frustrations for the patient and their family is perceived inefficiencies of care – the delays involved when they fear that any mistake may be the factor that causes them to lose a leg. This is not just the hours spent waiting for transport, or to be seen in clinic, but the days or weeks lost waiting for chiropody appointments, hospital referrals or cross-referrals. A decision to undertake an angiogram or an angioplasty is likely to be followed by a week's wait even in the best units, and a week is a long time to wait if you have an ischaemic foot. In less coordinated centres, the wait may be very much longer if it requires formal referral to another clinic and another consultant.

The delay which must be most difficult to accept is the time that lapses between a decision being made to undertake an amputation and the operation being done. The patient will want it done immediately, but they may have to wait for 2 weeks, and sometimes longer. But the speed of the process after surgery is even slower, with 3–4 weeks elapsing before they go home, and 3–4 months before they approach greater independence with the use an artificial limb. The whole process – from the development of the ulcer to the provision of a prosthesis – may take 2 years, and that means 2 years of immobility, dependence, fear and frustration in someone whose overall health and life expectancy are not good.

THE ROLE OF THE MULTIDISCIPLINARY CLINIC

Coordination of care

The main value of a multidisciplinary clinic is that it brings together the skills of different professionals such that they work most effectively in promoting the healing of established ulcers. Because they work together, some of the delays inherent in the process are eliminated. They also learn from each other in an area of clinical care where most of us start ignorant and untaught.

Most clinics in the UK are managed by a consultant physician, and if there is a single discipline which is not an immediate part of the team it is vascular surgery. Most will have tried to run combined clinics with surgeons but will have found that it is not cost-effective for two consultants to do a clinic together: one does the clinic and the other gets bored. The best solution is to arrange for the two consultants to run their own clinics – the diabetic foot clinic and the vascular clinic – in parallel, so that informal cross-referral is possible.

Education

The staff of the clinic refine their own knowledge and attitudes and are in an ideal position to coordinate education. This should be directed primarily at professional staff – doctors, community nurses, hospital nurses and chiropodists. On the basis of their educational role they should establish a network for easy and rapid advice and referral.

Research

The multidisciplinary clinic acts as the necessary focus for undertaking the research which is desperately needed. All aspects of care require further evaluation, as do techniques currently used for prevention. Research should be based on randomized prospective controlled trials.

Failings of the multidisciplinary service

The service is nearly always clinic (hospital) based and although this provides the most effective coordination of skills, it involves inconvenience to the patient and their carer. Moreover, it results in a barrier being created between the specialist team and those in primary care who are responsible for much of the day-to-day management. This needs to be recognized and efforts made to improve communication. There is a place for developing parallel outreach services, even though these should not replace the central clinic which should remain the base for urgent referrals.

Perhaps the greatest failing of the multidisciplinary service is its failure to make an impact on the delays which occur once an amputation has been performed. It is at this stage that the care of the patient becomes devolved to a separate team of physiotherapy and rehabilitation staff, which is especially true if the rehabilitation centre is based at a different hospital. It is possible that the process could be made better if closer coordination was achieved.

THE FUTURE

Prevention of foot ulcers

In the future it is hoped that the overall prevalence of significant vascular disease and neuropathy will be reduced in diabetes and that this will lead to a decline in ulceration. In the meantime greater awareness among patients and professionals of the foot which is 'at risk' will lead to more effective early management. However, the real breakthrough will come only when it is possible to reverse the process of atherosclerosis.

Coordination of care

Great improvements in outcome will be made if multidisciplinary services are established where they do not exist and achieve greater prominence where they do. They should act as a focus for urgent assessment of all ulcers and for the coordinated management in the community. Continued attempts should be made to develop education programmes – primarily targeted at professionals – and to improve communication.

In the hospitals there is a need for better communication between different professional units, and consideration should be given to the establishment in each hospital of a defined ward area in which all who require admission for ulcers are managed, as well as all amputations for diabetes and all those undergoing the process of rehabilitation. In this way it will be possible to deploy most effectively the many different professional skills required.

The St Vincent Declaration

The Declaration encompasses a list of targets for the management of diabetes that was formulated by representatives of the International Diabetes Federation and the World Health Organization in 1988. Although the time scale of the original Declaration was unrealistic (probably deliberately so), the principle has been adopted by many governments. The aim in this field is to reduce amputations of the leg by 50%.

However, our own evidence is that our overall amputation rate has remained unchanged for the last 10 years, at between six and eight a year. It seems unlikely that specialist clinics can refine their service still further in order to improve outcome to this extent. If the target of the St Vincent Declaration is achievable at all in a country like the UK given the current state of knowledge, then it can only be done by further coordination of resources such that all people with a diabetic foot ulcer have immediate access to a multidisciplinary service. We calculate that only one quarter of all such cases in our town are managed in the specialist clinic designed for them.

14 Practical guide to the management of lesions of the diabetic foot

GENERAL PRINCIPLES

There are many different types of ulcer and different ulcers require individual approaches to management. However, there are some general principles which apply to all. They take a long time to heal and many persist for months and even indefinitely. If they become complicated, there is an ever-present risk of amputation.

1. Refer all ulcers, by telephone, for expert assessment by a local multidisciplinary specialist unit – if such a unit exists.
2. Determine whether infection, ischaemia or neuropathy is the dominant problem.
3. If there is any sign of infection, treat the ulcer with an effective broad-spectrum antibiotic regimen immediately. Continue antibiotic therapy longer than usual, and at least until a formal management plan has been evolved.
4. Arrange for any ulcer to be dressed daily – by the patient, the family or a professional.
5. Advise the patient to rest the foot as much as possible in the early stages, and at least until a formal management plan has been evolved.
6. Arrange to review the ulcer at regular intervals and before any antibiotic course expires, in order to determine further action.
7. Remember that lesions which occur in an ischaemic leg are the ones which are most likely to deteriorate, leading to gangrene and amputation. If in doubt, refer early.
8. Remember that people with one complication of diabetes are likely to have others. For example, 40% of those who present with an ulcer and who were not previously known to have diabetes, will have retinopathy at the time of diagnosis.
9. Remember that people who have one ulcer are very likely to have another: of the 50% who survive 3 years after their first major amputation for diabetes, a fifth will lose the other leg as well. When any one ulcer has healed, it is essential to take steps to prevent recurrence. These steps include regular review, chiropody, education programme and the provision of fitted footwear.
10. In general, professionals believe that ulcers are healed by choosing specific antibiotics or specific dressings, but this is probably wrong. A major factor which hastens healing in the majority of cases is the commitment of the person caring for it.

SUGGESTED APPROACHES TO MANAGEMENT OF INDIVIDUAL LESIONS

The following suggestions are made for the best management of foot ulcers in primary and secondary care. In a field where there are few defined protocols, it must be accepted that guidelines such as these are based on personal experience and it is inevitable that personal experience is limited.

Furthermore, the following suggestions for the management of foot ulcers are made without any consideration being given to the patient, their social and other medical problems, or to local circumstances. It is accepted that in many cases the suggestions made below may have to be tempered by the need to consider other aspects of care. No mention is made of the effort that must be put into explanation and education – and yet these are obviously essential for the care of the person with an established ulcer, as well as for the prevention of any recurrence.

Case 1

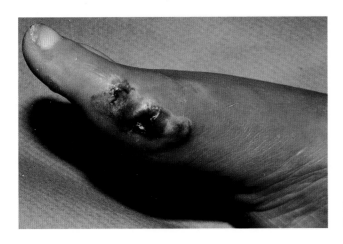

Case 1 The occurrence of gangrene indicates critical ischaemia.

HISTORY

The patient first noticed a blister 5 days earlier. It has got steadily worse, but is painless.

VISUAL ASSESSMENT

There is infection present in the area of necrosis, but the dominant problem is one of critical ischaemia – indicated by the gangrene (blackness) as well as by the smooth, shiny redness of the skin of the rest of the foot.

CLINICAL EXAMINATION

Document the degree of macrovascular disease and, in particular, determine whether the pulses are palpable higher in the leg. If the popliteal is missing but the femoral is palpable, there is a possibility that a revascularization procedure (angioplasty or bypass surgery) may help.

IMMEDIATE ACTION

Telephone to arrange a consultation within 24 hours. Prescribe broad-spectrum antibiotics (e.g. co-amoxiclav, or ofloxacin and metronidazole).

WOUND MANAGEMENT

Choice of dressings is unlikely to affect outcome. The wound should simply be cleaned daily and kept covered with a non-adherent dressing.

SPECIALIST CONSIDERATIONS

Specialist management would include early angiography to determine if the blood supply to the foot could be improved.

OUTCOME

It is probable that this leg will be lost. The complication of such a trivial lesion by gangrene indicates that the leg is critically ischaemic: the lesion will not heal, the infection will spread and so will the gangrene.

THE OTHER FOOT

A person with a foot like this is very likely to develop a pressure sore on the other foot while immobilized at home or in hospital. To lose one leg is a disaster, but for most patients, the thought of losing both is worse than that of dying. As there is more chance of saving the other foot, it should receive just as much care and attention as this one – if not more.

Case 2

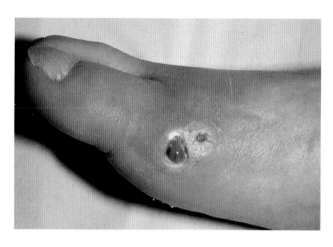

Case 2 If a neuroischaemic ulcer is painful, it is probably infected.

HISTORY

The ulcer has been present on this man's foot for 6 months and has persisted despite regular dressings. It was previously painless but has been hurting for three or four days.

VISUAL ASSESSMENT

The thin, red, hairless skin is typical of combined ischaemia and peripheral neuropathy: the man has a 'neuroischaemic' ulcer. The onset of pain suggests secondary infection, even though the signs of cellulitis are minimal, but this is confirmed by the appearance of exudate.

CLINICAL EXAMINATION

If the movement of the big toe squeezes out more exudate, it is probable that the joint is involved. Assess the degree of macrovascular disease by examining the femoral and popliteal arteries.

IMMEDIATE ACTION

Telephone to arrange for the ulcer to be reviewed within a few days. Start oral antibiotics with a broad spectrum and good bone penetration (e.g. co-amoxiclav; ofloxacin with metronidazole or clindamycin), in case there is osteomyelitis.

WOUND MANAGEMENT

Choice of dressings is unlikely to affect outcome. The ulcer should be cleaned daily and covered with a non-adherent dressing.

SPECIALIST CONSIDERATIONS

Plain X-ray will identify bone infection if it is obvious. The role of revascularization will be considered and an angiogram performed. If the blood supply to the foot cannot be improved, the only treatment is with continued antibiotics and simple measures. Attempts to eradicate bone infection by local surgical intervention would carry the risk of the wound not healing.

OUTCOME

If the blood supply cannot be improved, the ulcer is likely to persist for months.

THE OTHER FOOT

The other foot is very much at risk, and must be protected.

Case 3

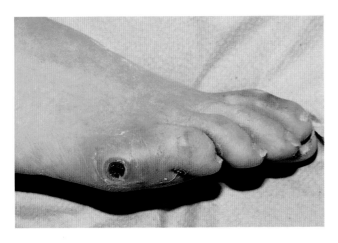

Case 3 Soft tissue infection showing signs of responding to antibiotic therapy.

HISTORY

This man had presented to another doctor 2 weeks earlier with painless cellulitis around the base of the fifth toe. It had been treated with a 5-day course of antibiotics.

VISUAL ASSESSMENT

There are signs of resolving soft tissue infection with flaking of the skin around the ulcer indicating earlier inflammation. This suggests that although the foot has an impaired blood supply, the ischaemia is not as critical as that in Case 2: if there is sufficient blood to mount an inflammatory response and to eradicate infection, there is likely to be enough to heal the ulcer.

CLINICAL EXAMINATION

Document the degree of macrovascular disease by feeling for the femoral, popliteal and pedal pulses.

IMMEDIATE ACTION

Telephone to arrange for the ulcer to be reviewed within a few days. Continue treatment with broad-spectrum antibiotics.

WOUND MANAGEMENT

Try to remove the slough by sharp debridement. Clean with saline or chlorhexidine. Follow this by application of a desloughing agent, such as a weak acid or a colloid/gel, and cover with a non-adherent dressing. Re-dress daily.

SPECIALIST CONSIDERATIONS

If the lesion is slow to heal, the main feature of specialist management would be to undertake angiography with a view to possible revascularization. In addition, a removable plaster boot may be provided to relieve any pressure on the ulcer from footwear.

OUTCOME

The ulcer should heal. However, the foot is ischaemic and hence the prognosis must be guarded: the foot may get worse.

THE OTHER FOOT

The other foot is at risk and should be protected.

Case 4

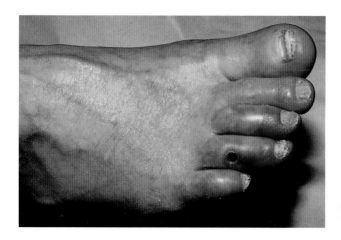

Case 4 Minor injuries should be taken seriously if the foot is severely ischaemic: they may easily lead to gangrene.

HISTORY

This man gives a long history of cardiovascular disease and has had previous arterial surgery in each leg for claudication. He had not noticed the ulcer and did not know how long it had been there.

VISUAL ASSESSMENT

The foot is obviously ischaemic, with skin which is thin and fragile. The nails are slow-growing and dystrophic, probably from mycotic infection. The lesion on the fourth toe has occurred because the fragile skin has been broken as a result of the normal trauma of wearing shoes. There is some adjacent bluish discolouration which is ominous. There is no obvious infection.

CLINICAL EXAMINATION

The possibility of further vascular reconstruction needs to be assessed.

IMMEDIATE ACTION

Telephone to arrange consultation within the next few days, or urgently if more extensive bluish discolouration suggests that the threat of gangrene is more marked.

WOUND MANAGEMENT

Simple hygiene and a daily dry dressing is all that is required. Povidone-iodine spray may be used to reduce the risk of infection by keeping the edges of the ulcer dry. Some would recommend that the ulcer was kept dry by exposing it as much as possible to the air. The foot should be protected by wearing soft and roomy slippers or shoes.

SPECIALIST CONSIDERATIONS

Further revascularization would be considered but, given the past history, it is likely that there is little that can be done.

OUTCOME

The outcome for the foot is poor. Other lesions are very likely and if any were to become infected, gangrene would be almost inevitable.

THE OTHER FOOT

The other foot is likely to be at just as great a risk.

Case 5

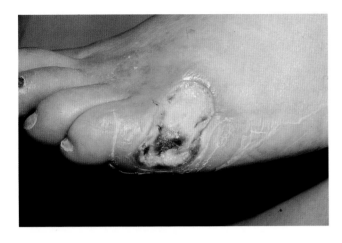

Case 5 The lack of any obvious inflammatory response indicates that early spontaneous healing is unlikely.

HISTORY

This old lady is blind, frail and lives in a rest home and does not know how long she has had this ulcer on her foot. It was first seen a week earlier when there was some surrounding cellulitis which was treated with antibiotics. It is painless.

VISUAL ASSESSMENT

The flaking of the skin shows that there has been preceding inflammation. This indicates that although the blood supply is poor, it was sufficient to mount an inflammatory response. The scab on the third toe is an indication, however, that the foot is generally ischaemic. The wound is covered by slough and soft eschar.

CLINICAL EXAMINATION

Document the degree of macrovascular disease by feeling for the arterial pulses in the leg and foot.

IMMEDIATE ACTION

There is no definite indication for continued antibiotics although secondary infection may occur at any stage. Telephone for specialist assessment within a few days.

WOUND MANAGEMENT

Sharp debridement should be followed by cleaning with saline or chlorhexidine. A desloughing agent, such as a weak acid or a colloid/gel should be applied, with the wound being re-dressed daily in the first instance.

SPECIALIST CONSIDERATIONS

Although revascularization would be considered despite her age and frailty, there is little else that can be done apart from keeping the ulcer under regular review.

OUTCOME

The ulcer is unlikely to heal and the defined policy of management should be to keep the patient symptom-free, to prevent secondary infection and to avoid mutilating surgery in someone whose overall prognosis is so poor.

THE OTHER FOOT

The other foot is very much at risk.

Case 6

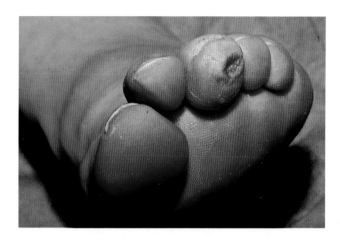

Case 6 Typical neuropathic ulcer.

HISTORY

This man found this ulcer when he picked off some hard skin from the end of his toe.

VISUAL ASSESSMENT

The appearances are of a classical neuropathic lesion: a clean, 'punched-out' ulcer with surrounding callus. There is no obvious infection and the general thickness of the skin suggests that the blood supply is well-preserved.

CLINICAL EXAMINATION

There will be reduced pin-prick sensation but the dorsalis pedis and posterior tibial pulses should be easily felt. If the toe looks swollen when viewed from above (see Case 7), the possibility of secondary bone infection should be considered.

IMMEDIATE ACTION

Telephone referral for specialist assessment within a few days. Advise the patient to rest the foot as much as possible and to avoid taking weight on the affected toe tip as much as possible.

WOUND MANAGEMENT

The callus around the margin should be pared away with a scalpel – with the object of leaving as thin a rim as possible. The ulcer should be cleaned with saline or chlorhexidine. It can be filled with a colloid/gel or an alginate preparation, before being covered with a non-adherent dressing. Dressings should be changed as often as is necessary to keep the wound base clean.

SPECIALIST CONSIDERATIONS

The main principle of management is the relief of pressure on the area, and this usually involves provision of a plaster boot. Arrangements should be made for repeated chiropody and for the provision of fitted footwear when the ulcer has healed.

OUTCOME

The median time to healing is 12 weeks, but the majority should heal without complication. The main risk is of secondary infection.

Case 7

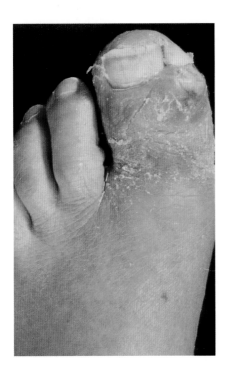

Case 7 The characteristic appearance of osteomyelitis in the toe.

HISTORY

This man noticed that his big toe had become red and swollen 10 days before the photograph was taken. He had been to the local Accident and Emergency Department and had been given a 5-day supply of antibiotics.

VISUAL ASSESSMENT

The appearances are typical of osteomyelitis: red and brawny, with sausage-like swelling of the toe and pus discharging from a wound on the medial aspect. The flaking of the skin suggests that the associated soft tissue infection has responded to the antibiotics.

CLINICAL EXAMINATION

The blood supply is usually well-preserved, but most have evidence of peripheral neuropathy.

IMMEDIATE ACTION

Start treatment with antibiotics effective against the most likely organisms (*Staphylococcus aureus* and anaerobic species), e.g. co-amoxiclav or ofloxacin with clindamycin or metronidazole. Telephone for an appointment within 2–3 days.

WOUND MANAGEMENT

The choice of dressings will not affect outcome. The toe should be simply kept clean and this will usually mean being re-dressed on a daily basis.

SPECIALIST MANAGEMENT

The diagnosis will usually be confirmed with a plain X-ray. Although surgery is the traditional recommendation, most would now use antibiotics alone. The foot should be rested as much as possible. Footwear should be provided when it has healed.

OUTCOME

The lesion should respond to prolonged (2–3 months) out-patient treatment with oral antibiotics, but the toe will be left shortened and deformed. This will put it at risk of secondary neuropathic ulceration.

Case 8

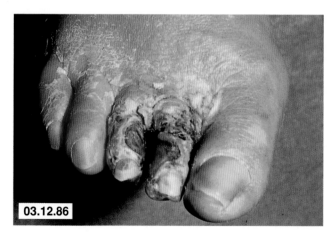

06.08.86

Case 8A Soft tissue infection of the toes, with possible underlying bone involvement.

HISTORY

The second and third toes on this lady's foot had always been partly fused but she had first noticed the sores 5 days earlier. They were painless.

VISUAL ASSESSMENT

The appearances are a bit uncertain. The swelling of the toes might be the result of the congenital deformity, or there may be bone infection present. The general condition of the foot is good, although the skin is a little thin and featureless, suggesting some degree of ischaemia.

CLINICAL EXAMINATION

It is important to decide on the degree of ischaemia; are the foot pulses palpable or not? If they are not, then the redness of the toes is a threatening sign and the foot should be referred for urgent review. If the pulses are palpable, the redness is more likely to be the result of infection.

IMMEDIATE ACTION

Telephone for urgent or early specialist assessment. Treat with antibiotics in case there is associated infection.

WOUND MANAGEMENT

The choice of dressings is unlikely to affect outcome. The foot simply needs to be kept clean and protected from trauma.

SPECIALIST CONSIDERATIONS

Plain X-ray and/or a labelled white cell scan would help resolve the question of bone infection. Angiography may be indicated if there is evidence of reduced peripheral blood flow.

OUTCOME

The degree of ischaemia proved more critical than initially expected. Revascularization proved impossible. The toes mummified, but the forefoot became secondarily infected and the onset of spreading gangrene led to amputation.

03.12.86

Case 8B The same foot 4 months later.

Case 9

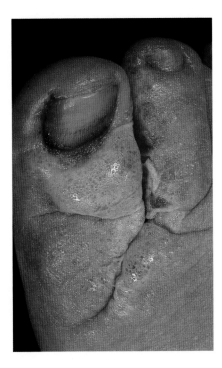

Case 9 Severe tinea pedis.

HISTORY

The blistering had been present for 4 days. The patient had been cleaning it with povidone-iodine solution which she had in the house.

VISUAL ASSESSMENT

The appearances are those of a severe mycotic infection (tinea pedis). Tinea pedis is normally seen as fissuring and flaking in the web space between the toes. Pathogenic bacteria can gain access to the tissues, and the occurrence of such infection in an ischaemic foot can lead to gangrene. The foot shown here does not look particularly ischaemic because the skin is thick and puffy, rather than thin and red.

CLINICAL EXAMINATION

The foot pulses should be palpable. Look out for signs of spreading bacterial cellulitis.

IMMEDIATE ACTION

Prescribe an antimycotic skin preparation, such as nystatin or an imidazole (e.g. miconazole). Advise the patient to wash her feet carefully twice daily, dry between the toes and then to apply the cream. Arrange to check that secondary infection has not occurred after 2–3 days. Oral terbinafine may be

considered. Specialist referral may not be necessary unless there are signs of complication.

OUTCOME

Complete healing is to be expected, although the infection may recur and the feet should be checked regularly.

THE OTHER FOOT

The other foot is likely to be infected also and both sides should be treated together.

Case 10

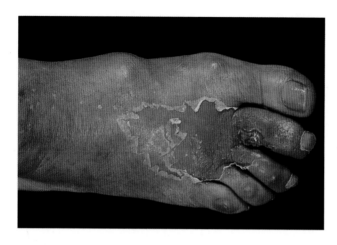

Case 10A Osteomyelitis of the toe.

HISTORY

This patient had presented to another doctor 2 weeks earlier with a swollen red foot, and had been treated with antibiotics. The discharge at the base of the second toe was first noted 10 days later. The foot was painless.

VISUAL ASSESSMENT

There are obvious signs of resolving soft tissue infection. However, the appearance of the second toe suggests that the bone is involved: it is swollen and sausage-like, and there is discharging pus. The organisms responsible must have gained access through a pre-existing break in the skin but it is not obvious in this case.

CLINICAL EXAMINATION

The blood supply is well-preserved, but there is likely to be evidence of peripheral neuropathy.

IMMEDIATE ACTION

Start treatment with antibiotics effective against the most likely organisms (*Staphylococcus aureus* and anaerobic species), e.g. co-amoxiclav or ofloxacin with clindamycin or metronidazole. Telephone for an appointment within 2–3 days.

WOUND MANAGEMENT

The choice of dressings will not affect outcome. The toe should be simply kept clean and bandaged.

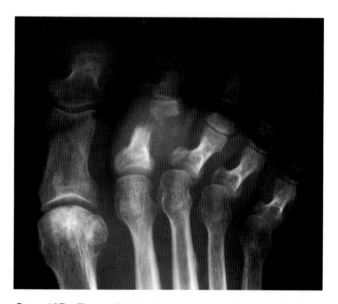

Case 10B The radiological appearance of osteomyelitis: interruption of the cortex of bone, with fragmentation.

SPECIALIST CONSIDERATIONS

The diagnosis of osteomyelitis should be confirmed with a plain X-ray. Although the infection should respond to prolonged treatment with effective antibiotic therapy, there is a case for considering amputation of the digit. Providing the blood supply to the foot is good, removal of the toe will lead to speedier resolution of the problem. Whether the foot is operated on or not, footwear will need to be provided.

OUTCOME

Complete healing can be expected, if the blood supply to the foot is good.

Case 11

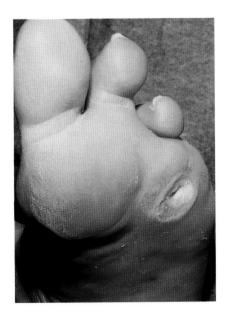

Case 11 Surgery to the foot can be complicated by neuropathic ulcers.

HISTORY

This man had previously had his fourth and fifth toes amputated. This ulcer was discovered at routine examination; he had not been aware of anything being wrong.

VISUAL ASSESSMENT

The appearance of the ulcer is typical of a neuropathic lesion caused, in this case, by increased pressure over the third metatarsal head. This pressure is at least partly the result of the mutilation caused by previous surgery. The skin of the surrounding foot does not look particularly ischaemic. There is no sign of infection.

CLINICAL EXAMINATION

The degree of macrovascular disease and of neuropathy should both be documented.

IMMEDIATE ACTION

Phone for early assessment. Advise the patient to keep his weight off the foot as much as possible.

WOUND MANAGEMENT

The ulcer simply needs to be kept clean and covered. There may be a case for packing bigger and deeper ulcers with a colloid/gel or with an alginate preparation.

SPECIALIST CONSIDERATIONS

Assuming that there is no suggestion of ischaemia, the main priority is to keep the ulcer clean and to allow it to heal by taking the weight off it with a Scotchcast boot or equivalent. This should be combined with regular chiropody to remove excessive callus. Fitted footwear should be provided once the lesion has healed.

OUTCOME

The median time to healing of neuropathic ulcers is 12 weeks, although those which are uncomplicated should heal in 1–2 months.

157

Case 12

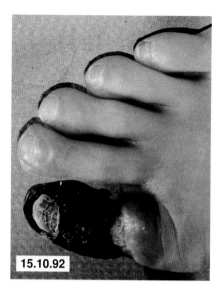

15.10.92

Case 12A Gangrene of a digit is usually the consequence of preceding soft tissue infection of a foot with underlying ischaemia.

HISTORY

This man is in his early 40s and has had diabetes for only 13 years. There is a strong family history of macrovascular disease and he has had an angioplasty for intermittent claudication. He continues to smoke cigarettes. He developed cellulitis of his big toe following a minor injury 3 weeks earlier and it has led to gangrene – despite being treated with antibiotics.

VISUAL ASSESSMENT

The gangrene is obvious but the toe is mummified and there is little exudate around the base. Any infection has been well treated.

CLINICAL EXAMINATION

The main priority in an ischaemic lesion is to determine whether there is any hope of improving the circulation to the foot by vascular reconstruction. Are the femoral, popliteal and foot pulses palpable?

IMMEDIATE ACTION

Telephone to arrange specialist review within 2–3 days.

WOUND MANAGEMENT

The aim is to prevent reinfection. The toe should be kept clean and dried thoroughly. Generally speaking, applications will neither hasten nor hinder healing.

SPECIALIST CONSIDERATIONS

If the blood supply to the foot is good, or can be improved by vascular reconstruction, then the toe should be amputated.

OUTCOME

The occurrence of gangrene in a young person has appalling prognostic significance. Not only is this man likely to lose his leg, from this or a later lesion, but he is also at risk of early death from myocardial infarction. This has to be borne in mind when determining management, although it will not help him to know it. In fact, this foot did not do well. Although the toe was amputated and the wound healed, he soon developed gangrene of adjacent toes.

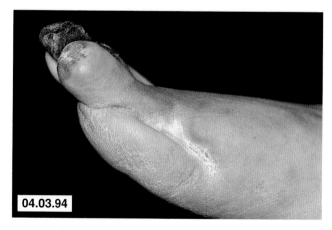

04.03.94

Case 12B The same foot 5 months later.

Case 13

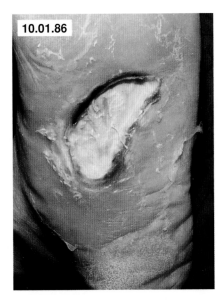

Case 13A Incision and drainage of an abscess has left an extensive indolent ulcer of the sole.

HISTORY

This lady had presented with an abscess under the sole and had had it incised by a general surgical team 3 weeks earlier.

VISUAL ASSESSMENT

The ulcer under the sole appears indolent with deep plantar fascia covered by slough. There is a surrounding rim of callus. The flaking of the skin indicates that previous inflammation has responded to antibiotic therapy. The foot is ischaemic, but it is a good sign that such significant soft tissue infection has already improved so much.

CLINICAL EXAMINATION

Examination of the pulses of the leg will determine both the extent of the vascular disease, as well as the possibility of vascular reconstruction.

IMMEDIATE MANAGEMENT

This should be referred by telephone for urgent assessment by a specialist team. Broad-spectrum antibiotics, such as co-amoxiclav, should be continued for as long as there are signs of infection.

WOUND MANAGEMENT

The wound on the sole should be managed by regular sharp debridement of the edge and base, associated with application of a weak acid or colloid/gel desloughing agent.

SPECIALIST CONSIDERATIONS

Ulcers of this type can prove to be very indolent and granulation tissue is slow to form over the deep fascia, even after it has been cleaned. Grafting does not help if the dermis has been completely destroyed. Angiography and vascular reconstruction may be considered, but the wound should heal – eventually.

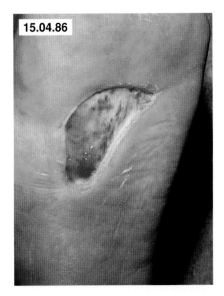

Case 13B After 3 months the ulcer is much cleaner and there are signs of healing.

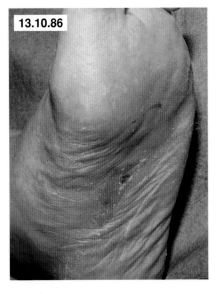

Case 13C Full healing occurred after 9 months, but some ulcers can take a lot longer.

Case 14

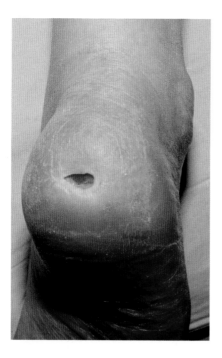

Case 14 If a small ulcer of the heel is painless, it is likely to be primarily neuropathic and it should heal. If it is painful, it is usually caused by small vessel thrombosis and the outlook is not so good.

HISTORY

The patient was not sure how this ulcer had started, but thinks it was from rubbing on a work boot. It was painless.

VISUAL INSPECTION

There is surrounding callus which suggests that this is primarily a neuropathic ulcer. If it was painful, it would indicate an ischaemic cause. The ulcer is relatively shallow – with the dermis being destroyed, but not the deeper tissues of the heel pad.

CLINICAL EXAMINATION

The presence of lost pin-prick sensation should be confirmed, and the degree of any associated vascular disease assessed.

IMMEDIATE ACTION

The immediate requirements are to pare away the callus from the edge, take the pressure off the ulcerated area and keep it clean.

WOUND MANAGEMENT

Regular sharp chiropody should be followed by cleaning with saline. If the wound is deeper, it may be packed with moistened alginate, but otherwise it should be sufficient to cover it with a simple non-adherent dressing. Dressings should be changed as often as is necessary to ensure that the ulcer remains clean.

SPECIALIST CONSIDERATIONS

A plaster boot may be used to take the weight off the area in the healing phase. This is an unusual site for neuropathic ulceration and it is probable that there is significant associated vascular disease.

OUTCOME

It should heal quickly.

THE OTHER FOOT

Both feet are likely to be at great risk and arrangements should be made for regular review. Fitted footwear should be considered.

Case 15

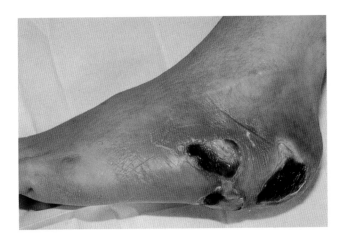

Case 15 Widespread soft tissue infection complicating a pressure sore on the heel.

HISTORY

This man had pre-existing severe peripheral neuropathy, and had developed a dry pressure sore on the outside of his heel when immobilized with a chest infection. It had become swollen and painful in the preceding 3 days.

VISUAL ASSESSMENT

The occurrence of pain in a neuropathic foot usually means infection, and in this case it is obvious. The portal of entry is the soft moist area above the eschar of the pre-existing ulcer on the heel. The infection has spread rapidly and has already caused extensive destruction.

IMMEDIATE ACTION

The patient should be referred for review as an emergency.

WOUND MANAGEMENT

The choice of dressing will not affect outcome. The wound should be cleaned and covered. If the wound smells, an activated charcoal dressing may be used, or metronidazole gel applied.

SPECIALIST CONSIDERATIONS

It is unlikely that the leg can be saved because the occurrence of the original pressure sore indicates that the foot is also relatively ischaemic. Broad-spectrum antibiotics should be given intravenously and local debridement undertaken. However, infection in this area can be impossible to eradicate and even if it can be, the tissues of the heel do not reform.

Angiography and vascular reconstruction should be considered before proceeding to any amputation.

THE OTHER FOOT

The other foot is at very great risk – especially if this leg is amputated and the patient is thus bedridden for any length of time.

OUTCOME

This leg was lost and the patient acquired a heel ulcer on the other leg during the recovery phase. That also became infected and that leg had to be amputated as well. Muscle weakness from neuropathy prevented any rehabilitation with prostheses, and he was left wheelchair-bound, totally dependent on others and severely depressed.

Case 16

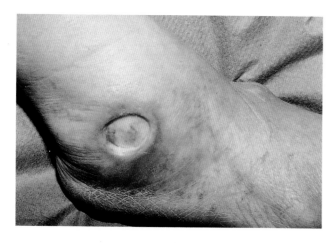

Case 16 An indolent ulcer showing little sign of healing.

HISTORY

This lady had rheumatoid arthritis as well as diabetes. This ulcer had been present and painless for 3 months despite regular dressings from the community nurse. It had been previously painless but had been hurting badly for a week.

VISUAL ASSESSMENT

The pain indicates infection and the absence of any obvious cellulitis indicates quite severe vascular disease. This is also reflected in the indolence of the ulcer itself: it shows little sign of healing.

CLINICAL EXAMINATION

Examination will confirm the presence of both vascular disease and neuropathy. Examination of the femoral and popliteal pulses will indicate if the patient may benefit from vascular reconstruction.

IMMEDIATE ACTION

Broad-spectrum antibiotics should be prescribed and the patient should be referred by telephone for specialist review within the next few days.

WOUND MANAGEMENT

The wound should be dressed daily, with a desloughing agent being applied. A colloid or gel should probably be chosen to pack the wound, rather than a weak acid cream. Such preparations swell as they absorb moisture and may relieve pain by compressing the base of the wound. The application should be covered by a non-adherent dressing.

SPECIALIST CONSIDERATIONS

Angiography and vascular reconstruction should be considered because there is little else that can be done. However, the combination of diabetes and rheumatoid arthritis suggests that the main problem is microvascular disease.

OUTCOME

If the ulcer has resulted from dominant microvascular disease, then the leg is not at particular risk of gangrene. On the other hand healing may be very slow, and the wound will be susceptible to recurrent infections. It may never heal.

Index

Age
  at amputation 3
  at death from gangrene 3
  complications of 20, 25
Alginates 111, 114, 118
Amputation 119–30
  above-knee 126
  below-knee 126
  complications of localized surgery 45, 122–4
  contraindications to 125
  costs 8, 142–3
  digit 60, 103, 120–3
  Gritti–Stokes 126
  indications for 120–1, 123–4
  mean age for 3
  outcome after 130
  phantom limb 129
  prevalence of 142
  prostheses 127–8
  psychological problems 129, 143
  ray excision 120, 124
  rehabilitation following 126–9
  seasonal variation 4
  secondary ulceration 124, 129–30
  survival after 8, 125, 130, 142
  Syme's operation 122
Anaerobic bacteria
  smell 37–8, 43, 116
  see also Microbiology
Anatomy 13–18
  blood supply 13–17
  bones and joints 13–15
  innervation 13, 17–18
Angiography
  digital subtraction imaging 62–3, 66
  indications for 61–2
  Seldinger technique 62
Angioplasty 63–5
  effectiveness 65
  stents 65
Anhidrosis 75, 90, 95
Antibiotics
  choice of 46–9
  osteomyelitis treatment of 43
  prophylactic 121
  topical 113–14, 118

Applications 105–18
  alginates 114
  growth factors 114
  hydrocortisone 114–15, 118
  topical antibiotics 113–14
  see also Cleaning agents, Desloughing agents, Dressings
Arterial surgery 62–7
  see also Ischaemia
Arteriovenous shunting 22, 55, 73–5, 92
  see also Autonomic neuropathy, Neuropathic osteoarthopathy
Atherosclerosis 20, 53–4
  see also Macrovascular disease
'At Risk' foot 19–30, 56–7, 75–9, 133–7
Autonomic neuropathy 23, 73–5, 90, 95
  anhidrosis 75, 90, 95
  arteriovenous shunting 73–5
  hair loss 75–6
  recognition 75–6
  vasomotor 73–5

Balance platform 73
Basement membrane thickening 21, 55
Bed sores, *see* Pressure sores
Biosthesiometer 77
Biphosphonates 87
Blisters 59, 92–3
Bone biopsy 42, 86
Bone infection, *see* Osteomyelitis
Bones, *see* Anatomy
Buerger's test 57-8
Bullosis diabeticorum 92–3
  see also Blisters
Burns and scalds 6, 15, 25, 27, 67, 70, 93

Callus, *see* Neuropathic ulceration
Candida albicans, see Tinea pedis
Capillaries, *see* Microvascular disease
Carers, *see* Family and carers
Cellulitis, *see* Soft tissue infection
Charcoal, activated 116, 118
Charcot deformity, *see* Neuropathic osteoarthropathy
Charcot, Jean-Martin 82
Charcot joint, *see* Neuropathic osteoarthropathy
Charcot neuropathic osteoarthropathy, *see* Neuropathic

osteoarthropathy
Chiropody 100–4, 125, 133
   nail care 100–1
   neuropathic callus 78, 102–3
   role of 103–4
   skin care 100
   see also Debridement
Classification of ulcers 32–3
   Meggit/Wagner 32
   Nottingham 32–3
Clawing of toes 24, 71, 75, 79
Cleaning agents 111, 113, 118
Corns 102
Costs 2, 8, 142–3
   duration of hospital stay 8
   footwear 139
   ulcer management 143
   see also Amputation

Death 2, 4, 9
Debridement 102–4, 109–12
   gentle 110–1
   sharp 110
   see also Chiropody, Desloughing agents, Eschar,
      Slough
Dermatitis artefacta 94
Dermatophytes, *see* Tinea pedis
Descriptions of ulcers 33–4
Desloughing agents 111–12, 118
   enzymatic 111–12
   gels/colloids 111–12
   hydrogen peroxide 111–12
   weak acids 111–12
Diabetic dermopathy 91
Digital subtraction imaging 62–3, 66
Doppler ultrasonography 59–60
Dressings 105–18
   absorbent 111, 115, 118
   activated charcoal 116, 118
   adverse effects of 113, 117
   compression bandaging 116
   gauze 115, 118
   hydrocolloids 111, 115–16, 118
   low adherent 115, 188
   paraffin tulle 111, 115, 118
   psychological aspects of 116
   purpose of 114–15
   semi-permeable film 111, 116, 118
   see also Applications
Duplex ultrasonography 60–1

Eczema 94–5
Education 6, 30
   adverse effects of 136
   multidisciplinary clinics and 144
   of people with diabetes 132–6
   of the profession 136–8
Eruptive xanthomata 91

Eschar 108–9
   see also Desloughing agents
Exudate 37, 116, 147

Family and carers 143
Flat feet 13, 71
Footwear
   Charcot neuropathic osteoarthropathy 79, 88, 138–9
   costs 139
   fitted 78–80, 88, 138–9
   ill-fitting 6, 25, 75, 79
   prevention of neuropathic ulceration 78–80, 138–9
   slippers 133

Gangrene
   amputation and 120, 124
   gas 37
   historical perspective 2–9
   infection secondary to 29, 39, 62
Gas-forming organisms 38, 43, 121
Gender factors 3, 20, 91
Glycaemic control 6
Grafts, *see* Skin, arterial surgery
Gram-negative bacteria, *see* Microbiology
Gram-positive bacteria, *see* Microbiology
Granulation tissue
   excessive 114–15
Granuloma annulare 91–2
Griseofulvin 98

Hands
   prayer sign 24–5
   signs of neuropathy 71, 75
Healing
   impaired 27–30
   process of 52–3, 106–8
   promotion of 135
   scab formation
Heels
   cracks 56, 100
   protection 9, 80, 138
Histology 42, 53–4
Hormone replacement therapy 55
Hotwater bottles, *see* Trauma
Hydrocortisone 114–15, 118
Hygiene 4, 48, 113
Hyperkeratosis, *see* Psoriasis, Neuropathic ulceration
Hyperlipidaemia 54, 91

Infarcts 56
Infection 35–48
   anhidrosis and 90, 95
   antibiotic choice 46–9
   gangrene and 29, 39, 62, 120
   gas-forming organisms 38, 43, 121
   microbiology 38–9, 43–8
   osteomyelitis 39–43
   pain and 38

soft tissue infection 37–9
subacute 37
treatment of 43–9
Inflammation 52–3
In-growing toenails 36, 96, 100
Ischaemia 51–68, 95
identification of 56–9
investigations 57–62
signs 28
treatment
arterial surgery 66
skin grafting 67–8
thrombolysis 66
see also Angioplasty
typical foot ulcers in 57–9
see also Angiography, Gangrene, Macrovascular
disease, Microvascular disease, Pathogenesis
Isotope scans
biphosphonate-labelled 87
leucocyte-labelled 42, 86

Joints
limited mobility of 24–5
normal 13
see also Clawing of toes
Joslin, Elliott 2

Lichen planus 92
Lisfranc's disarticulation 83

Macrovascular disease
atherogenesis 20–1, 53–4
risk factors 54–5
see also Smoking
Magnetic resonance imaging (MRI) 86
Martorell's ulcer 95
Microbiology 38–9, 43–8
anaerobic bacteria 38–9, 114
colonization 95
gas-forming organisms 38, 43, 121
Gram-negative bacteria 38–9
Gram-positive bacteria 38–9, 43
sensitivity to antibacterial agents 47
swab technique 46–7
see also Antibiotics, Infection
Microvascular disease 20–2, 55–6
see also Arteriovenous shunting, Basement membrane
thickening
Motor neuropathy, *see* Neuropathy
Multidisciplinary clinic
failings of 144
role of 143–4
Mycological infections
nail 95–8, 101
see also Tinea pedis, Tinea unguium

Nails
care of 100–1, 134

clipping 97
dystrophy 57, 95, 101
mycological infections 97–8
Necrobiosis lipoidica 37–8, 90–2
Nephropathy 56
Neuropathic osteoarthropathy 23, 82–8, 120
acute phase 42, 83, 85
arteriovenous shunting 83
cup and ball deformity 82–3
investigations 86–7
Lisfranc's disarticulation 83
management 87–8
pathogenesis 83–5
sclerotic phase 83–4
signs 85
sucked pencil deformity 82–3
ray excision 120
see also Footwear
Neuropathic ulceration 28, 71–2, 102–4
management of 80–1
median time to healing 81
prevention 78–80
see also Amputation, Chiropody, Footwear, Heels,
Plastercasts
Neuropathy 69–88
arched foot 13, 24, 71–2, 75
clawing of toes 24, 71–2, 75, 78
investigation 76-8
motor 24, 71–3, 135
muscle wasting 24, 71, 75
painful 70–1
peripheral sensory 22, 24, 70–1, 134–5
proprioception 73
Von Frey monofilaments 76
see also Autonomic neuropathy, Neuropathic
ulceration, Neuropathic osteoarthropathy

Onychauxis 97–8
Onychia 97
Onychogryphosis 97–8, 134
Onycholysis 97
Onychomycosis 97–8
Orthoses, *see* Footwear
Osteomyelitis 8
Charcot deformity and 41–5
identification 33, 39–42
investigations for 41–2
management of 43–9
radiological signs 40–1
treatment 43, 49

Pain 37–9, 56, 59, 70–1
Paronychia 96
Pathogenesis 19–30
infection 36
ischaemia 20–2, 53–5
neuropathic osteoarthropathy 23, 83–5
neuropathy 23–6, 70–7

Pathogenesis *contd*
  osteomyelitis 39
Pedobarography 77–8
Phantom limb 129
Plastercasts
  Scotchcasts 67, 80–1
  total contact 81
Plethysmography, toe 60
Prayer sign 25
Pressure sores 26, 36, 137–8
Prevention of foot ulcers 131–40
  'At Risk' foot 133–7
  chiropody 133, 137
  heel protection 9, 80, 138
  see also Education, Footwear
Prostheses 127–8
Psoriasis 92–3, 98
Psychological aspects
  amputation 120, 126, 129
  foot ulceration 143
  wound management 116

Rashes, *see* Skin disorders
Referral
  barriers to 28–30, 143
  delays in 9
  letters 33
  times 135
Rehabilitation, *see* Amputation
Retinopathy 22, 56
Risk factors 20, 54, 77–8

Saint Vincent declaration 144
Scab formation 107
Scotchcasts, *see* Plastercasts
Seldinger technique 62
Shin ulcers 27, 36, 60, 68, 94–5, 108
Shoes, *see* Footwear
Skin
  care of 100
  cracks 56, 100
  dry 22–3, 74–5, 77, 90
  see also Skin disorders, Skin grafting, Tinea pedis
Skin disorders 89–98
  anhidrosis 90
  bullosis diabeticorum 92–3
  dermatitis artefacta 94
  diabetic dermopathy 91
  eczema 94–5
  eruptive xanthomata 91
  granuloma annulare 92
  lichen planus 92
  Martorell's ulcer 95
  necrobiosis lipoidica 38, 90–2
  psoriasis 92–3, 98
  purpura 94–5
  rashes 91, 94–5
  vasculitis 94

Skin grafting 67–8, 114
  see also Ischaemia
Slough 108–9
  see also Debridement, Desloughing agents
Smell, *see* Anaerobic bacteria
Smoking 20–1, 54–5, 132
Social factors 29–30
Soft tissue infection 37–9
  gas-forming organisms 38, 43, 121
  treatment of 46–9
Stents 65
Stroke 61, 63–6
Swab technique 46–7
  see also Microbiology
Sweating, loss of 23, 75, 90

TCO_2, *see* Transcutaneous oxygen tension
Terbinafine 98
Thrombolysis 60
Tinea pedis 6, 26, 29, 33–4, 36, 114
  dermatophytosis 95–7
  yeasts 96–7
Tinea unguium 97–8
Transcutaneous oxygen tension 60
Trauma 20, 25–6, 70–1, 93–4
  footwear 6, 36, 75, 79
  hotwater bottles 6, 93, 135
Trichophytons, *see* Tinea pedis, Tinea unguium

Ulcers
  case histories 145–62
  glycaemic control and 6
  healing process 52–3, 106–8
  in perspective 141–4
  kissing 28, 59
  neuroischaemic 28, 33, 57–9, 73, 103
  prevalence of 20, 142
  see also Applications, Blisters, Classification, Cleaning agents, Descriptions, Dressings, Heels, Infection, Ischaemia, Neuropathic ulceration, Pathogenesis, Prevention of foot ulcers, Referral, Shin ulcers, Tinea, Trauma
Ultrasonography
  duplex 60–1
  hand-held Doppler 60

Vasculitic rash 94
Vasculopathy, *see* Ischaemia

Walking plasters, *see* Plastercasts
Wound healing, *see* Healing

Xanthomata, eruptive 91
X-rays, *see* Angiography, Angioplasty, Computed tomography, Digital subtraction imaging, Osteomyelitis

Yeasts, *see* Tinea pedis, Tinea unguium